# Robotic Surgery

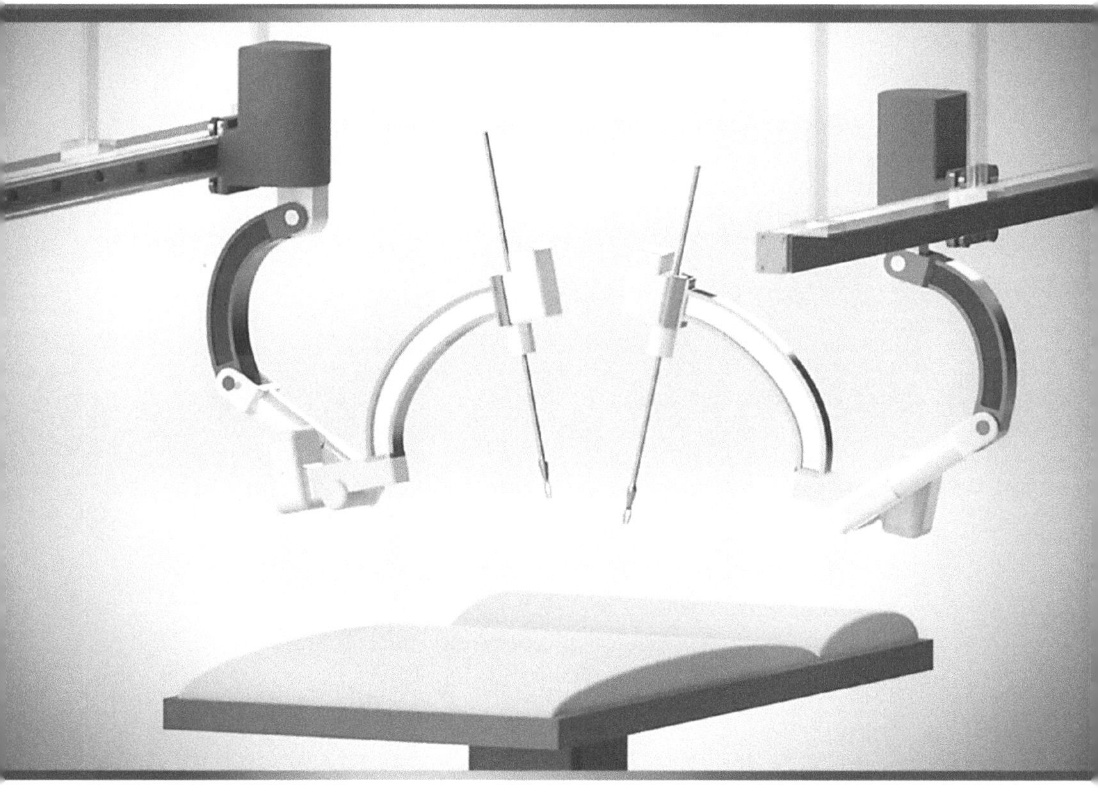

# Robotic Surgery

## Smart Materials, Robotic Structures, and Artificial Muscles

Mohsen Shahinpoor
Siavash Gheshmi

CRC Press
Taylor & Francis Group
Boca Raton London New York

CRC Press is an imprint of the
Taylor & Francis Group, an **informa** business

**Robotic Surgery: Smart Materials, Robotic Structures, and Artificial Muscles**

First published in 2015 by Pan Stanford Publishing Pte. Ltd.

Published 2022 by CRC Press
Taylor & Francis Group
6000 Broken Sound Parkway NW, Suite 300
Boca Raton, FL 33487-2742



ISBN-13: 978-981-4316-23-1 (hbk)



**British Library Cataloguing-in-Publication Data**
A catalogue record for this book is available from the British Library.

**Visit the Taylor & Francis Web site at**
**http://www.taylorandfrancis.com**

**and the CRC Press Web site at**
**http://www.crcpress.com**

*To the memory of my parents,*
*Zarrin Taj and Aliasghar*

*—Mohsen Shahinpoor*

*To my parents,*
*Farahnaaz and Akbar*

*—Siavash Gheshmi*

# Contents

# Preface

Robotic surgery is one of the fields where medicine and technology come together to enhance the quality of life. There are many books on robotic surgery that are specifically written for surgeons to describe how to use a robotic system to perform a surgical intervention. The focus of these books is purely medicine. There was a lack of a technical book that covers both the engineering design aspect of robotic surgical systems and how surgeons can benefit from them, which was our motivation to write the first textbook on robotic surgery that covers both medical and engineering aspects of this emerging field of remote surgical operations, and also offer homework problems to further enhance the underlying educational endeavors. *Robotic Surgery with Smart Materials, Robotic Structures and Artificial Muscles* is respectfully presented to the researchers and students of various disciplines of engineering and medicine to further expand their understanding of the field. This book also answers the need for a comprehensive review of medical robotics and their applications. The material presented in this text book is the result of collaborations of engineers and surgeons.

This book is the first textbook in robotic surgery that discusses the integration of smart multi-functional soft and biomimetic materials with robotic end effectors to provide haptic and tactile feedback to surgeons. It is also the first textbook in robotic surgery that comes with a solutions manual which makes it useful as a supplement to faculty members teaching many different programs and courses such as robotics, medical devices, surgical interventions and many more.

This book can be adapted by professors to teach the subject, used by graduate students and researchers to enable them to further employ their creativity and knowledge and by undergraduates to simply get an excellent grasp of this exciting field. It is also useful to those interested in the field for self-study. The background required to this book is college-level mathematics, matrix analysis, geometry and medical/surgical terminologies.

We acknowledge the collaboration and help of a number of surgeons who have contributed towards completing this book. In particular Dr. David Soltanpour, MD, Ophthalmologist and Micro-surgeon at New York Eye and Ear Infirmary, Dr. Alireza Ghaffarieh, Ocular Pathology Fellowship, Department of Ophthalmology and Visual Science at University of Wisconsin, Madison as well as Michelle Toder, MD, Bariatric Robotic Surgeon at Eastern Maine Medical Center.

**Mohsen Shahinpoor**
**Siavash Gheshmi**

# Foreword

Robotic surgery has already created a paradigm shift in medical surgical procedures and will continue to expand to all surgical and microsurgical procedures. There is no doubt that in doing so robotic surgical systems, such as the da Vinci surgical system, will become much more intelligent and sophisticated with the integration, implementation, and synergy of new intelligent material systems that will make surgical tools and equipment more functional and more intelligent in biomimetic sensing and actuation and kinesthetic interaction with organs during robotic surgery.

The current robotic surgical systems evolved from laparoscopic surgical procedures and made it possible for surgeons to perform surgery away from the patient, with much more concentration and ease. However, what was lost in this transition by the surgeons was the feeling sensation of tissues and organs and the kinesthetic force feedback during surgery. It is interesting to note that even during laparoscopic surgery surgeons can still feel and sense the tissues and organs they are handling and operating on with laparoscopic/endoscopic tools and feel the kinesthetic forces at work. However, kinesthetic force feedback was replaced with visual feedback during robotic surgery. It is to be noted that some of this kinesthetic force feedback was lost in the transition from open to laparoscopic surgery due to trocar friction and varying lever arms, anyway. However, using smart materials such as ionic polymer metal composites (IPMCs) and appropriate calibration and tuning, one may be able to recover the kinesthetic force feedback during surgery. IPMCs are great for such robotic force feedback applications because they work perfectly well in the wet human body environment and generate a millivolt-level sensing signal for kinesthetic force feedback. We believe that considering IPMCs for haptic and kinesthetic force feedback is novel. This topic is covered in Chapter 5.

Chapter 1 introduces surgical robots and their general or specific configurations for various types of surgery. Chapter 2 presents direct kinematics, inverse kinematics, and workspace considerations for surgical robots. Chapter 3 covers a thorough discussion and description of ophthalmic surgical robots and systems for performing microrobotic surgery. Chapter 4 presents a number of novel designs on deployable laparoscopic robotic surgical systems with 3D flexibility and orientational capabilities during robotic surgery. Chapter 5 discusses applications of intelligent materials and artificial muscles in robotic surgery in connection with haptic, tactile, and kinesthetic force feedback to surgeons during robotic surgery. Chapter 6 presents a summary of the coverage, as well as conclusions and future prospects for robotic surgery. The book ends with a large number of references, an appendix of MATLAB codes used, an authors' index, and a detailed subject index.

# Chapter 1

# Introduction to Surgical Robots' General Configurations

## 1.1 History of Robotics

Malone (1978) mentions that Aristotle was the first to discuss the concept of automation as a means to avoid the need for servants. The first versions of robots mostly consisted of clocks, such as the clepsydra (the water clock that measures time through a graduated flow of liquid passing through a small opening [Bedini, 1962]), pioneered by Ctesibius of Alexandria (c. 270 BC) (Rosheim, 1994), subsequently followed by self-moving machines or automatons. The use of automatons was also related to clocks, such as the case of 1497, where two bell-striking giants decorated the clock tower in Piazza San Marco, Venice. Later in history, cuckoo clocks emerged and gained popularity, especially in Germany. Leonardo da Vinci did considerable and notable work on robotics, mostly found in his renowned book *Codex Atlanticus*. Da Vinci planned to build an *anthrobot*, though a proper source of energy or the necessary high-precision part manufacturing to build such a robot did not exist in contemporary technology (Pires, 2000). The invention of the textile machine in 1801 by Joseph Jacquard was one of the catalysts and symbols of the Industrial Revolution, which took place in 1750–1850. The first industrial robot was designed by Seward Babbitt in 1892. This was a motorized crane with a gripper for the removal of

*Robotic Surgery: Smart Materials, Robotic Structures, and Artificial Muscles*
Mohsen Shahinpoor and Siavash Gheshmi

ISBN 978-981-4316-23-1 (Hardcover), 978-981-4463-51-5 (eBook)
www.panstanford.com

ingots from a furnace. Tesla (1898) gave his precious contribution in robotics through his patented remotely controlled device, the first of its kind, among many other inventions that are products of his work.

The word "robot" seems to have first become popular when the Czech playwright Karel Capek's play, entitled "Rossum's Universal Robots" (RUR), was first performed in Paris, France, in the 1920s. In that play, small, artificial, and anthropomorphic creatures strictly obeyed their master's orders. In Czech and Russian these creatures were called *robotnic*, from *robota*, which are the Czech and Russian words for "drudgery" and "hard work." "Robotics" as a term, on the other hand, was introduced later, in 1942, by Isaac Asimov in the story "Runaround," in which the author also submitted the laws of robotics (Asimov, 2012). These laws can be summarized as follows:

(a) Law 1: A robot may not harm a human being or, through inaction, allow a human being to come to harm.
(b) Law 2: Robots must obey orders given by humans, except those that would conflict with the higher-order laws.
(c) Law 3: Robots must protect their own existences as long as such protection does not conflict with the higher-order laws.

Asimov's laws have found real-world applications, particularly in modern surgical robots. According to Shahinpoor's (2011) book entitled *Intelligent Robotic Systems: Modeling & Simulation*, a robot is a reprogrammable, multifunctional manipulator designed to move materials, parts, tools, or specialized devices through variable programmed motions for a variety of tasks. This definition covers a broad spectrum of robot manipulators, and within this definition, there are different classes of robots. These classes include the following:

1. *Automated or flexible manufacturing.* These "industrial" robots are employed in a wide range of manufacturing processes, including parts assembly and inspection, materials handling, welding, and materials painting.
2. *Remote exploration.* This class of robotic manipulators is designed to survive in environments that humans cannot tolerate. These robots can be used to explore the unknown, from the edge of our solar system to the depths of the earth's oceans.

3. *Prosthetic and biomedical fields.* Robotic technology and its accompanying sensor technology can be teamed up with one another to provide prosthetic limbs with touch sensation. Miniature robots under a surgeon's control can probe the human body to operate on patients from within their bodies.
4. *Hazardous material handling.* Robots in this class have been employed to remove bombs and handle hazardous materials.
5. *Service.* Some present uses for service robots include security, janitorial, mail delivery, fire sentry, firefighter, and voice-commanded errand robots. The use of service robots will increase as technology progresses and manufacturing costs fall.

Westinghouse conceived two robots in 1940 that utilized electric motors for comprehensive body motion and, among other activities, imitated human and animal behaviors. One exhibited human behavior by dancing and counting to 10. The other exhibited animal behavior by walking, standing on its hind legs, and barking. The year 1946 marks the beginning of the computer age, with the introduction of several inventions that will be expounded on herein. George Devol invented a playback device used in controlling machines through the introduction of a magnetic process recorder. J. Presper Eckert and John Mauchly are credited for building the first computer that used electronic components, electronic numerical integrator and computer (ENIAC), while the first digital computer was conceived at the Massachusetts Institute of Technology (MIT) and was called Whirlwind. Norbert Wiener published a book, *Cybernetics*, that described the concept of communications and control in mechanical, biological, and electronic systems (Diodato, Prasad, and Klingensmith, 2004).

The invention of the transistor in 1948 marked the start of a new era of inventions and advents in computing, which expedited the development of robots that functioned in conjunction with this new generation of computers. Raymond Goetz invented an articulated arm equipped with a teleoperator for the Atomic Energy Commission (AEC) in 1951. Devol and Engelberger were the first to develop a programmable robot in 1954, called Unimate, and linked it to the term "universal automaton" (please refer to the previous reference for the term "automaton"). Engelberger went on to establish Unimation, the world's first robot company.

The first commercial robot was made available in the market by Planet Corporation in 1959. In 1960, Condec Corporation purchased Unimation and began development of the Ultimate Robot System. In 1962, General Motors started equipping production lines in Trenton, New Jersey, with robots. By 1964, MIT, Stanford University, and the University of Edinburgh had laboratories devoted to research on artificial intelligence. Hughes Aircraft developed the remotely controlled Mobots, specifically designed for use in "environments beyond (human) capacity and for tasks beyond (human) capability" (Asimov and Frenkel, 1985), including construction, chemical testing, and interaction in nuclear reactor environments. In 1968, researchers at the Stanford Research Institute developed Shakey, a robot equipped with visual capabilities. In 1970, Stanford University introduced an electrically powered robotic arm. In 1973, Richard Hohn designed the first commercial minicomputer-controlled robot called T3, or the Tomorrow Tool. In 1974, Scheinman incorporated the company called Vicarm, with the aim to market an industrial version of the computer-controlled robotic arm that was developed by the Stanford research group. This robotic arm was to be used by NASA during the Viking space probes. In 1978, Unimation, under continuous support by General Motors, developed the Programmable Universal Machine for Assembly (PUMA).

The computer industry experienced the beginning of sustained success during the 1980s, the profits of which were also conveyed to the robotic industry. Fujitsu Fanuc Co. started the first completely automated factory in 1980, while a large number of new robotics companies were entering the market. By 1990, just 40 Japanese and 12 American companies were controlling a $170 billion industry due to numerous purchases of small companies that these companies made. These robotic companies made improvements on the human–robot interface, which resulted in the development of the first visual-servo-controlled systems. On the other hand, feedback systems were continuously being improved, which, as a result, sparked interest in a novel market for robotics: medicine.[1] The first tests of robotics in medicine were successful, which encouraged a wave of innovations and enthusiasm, stemming from the belief that the convergence of robotics with medicine would yield extraordinary results in the future (Patel, 2008).

---

[1]http://www.cs.bham.ac.uk/research/robotics/cbbc/history.php

Computer Motion and Intuitive Surgical were the two major companies in the development and marketing of surgical robotic systems, until Intuitive Surgical purchased Computer Motion in 2003.[2,3] Computer Motion (Goleta, CA), founded in 1989 by Yulun Wang, PhD, introduced a voice-controlled robotic arm, AESOP®, in 1993 for use in laparoscopy. In 1994, AESOP® was the first surgical robot to be cleared by the Food and Drug Administration (FDA), while a further generation of AESOP®, AESOP® 2000, became the first voice-controlled robot to be cleared by the FDA in 1996. Another product by Computer Motion, the ZEUS® Robotic Microsurgical System, was introduced in 1998 and consists of a slave robot with three robotic arms and a master surgeon's console, from which the surgeon telemanipulates the robotic arms to conduct surgery. Intuitive Surgical (Sunnydale, CA) was founded in 1995 by Frederic Moll, MD; Robert Younge; and John Freund, MD, and was based on technology developed at the Stanford Research Institute. The most important product of Intuitive Surgical is the da Vinci® Surgical System, consisting of a slave robotic system that performs surgery through four manipulator arms and a surgeon console that houses a surgeon as master of the surgery. The da Vinci® system is currently the most widely used system in general surgery and is also the first robotic system to be used in cardiac interventions: in a mitral valve procedure in 1998 in Paris (Carpentier et al., 1998) by Alain F. Carpentier, MD, and in a coronary artery bypass graft (CABG) procedure performed by Friedrich Mohr, MD, in Leipzig in the same year (Mohr et al., 1999).

## 1.2 Introduction to Robotic Surgery

Human surgery is under constant change. Its development is led by the need for more efficient practices that require minimal incision on bodies and organs of patients, more precision, reduced hospitalization time, and expedited recovery and healing. Though improvement on manual procedures has yielded successively better results, these are merely marginal and do not reflect the real need for effective techniques. The future of surgery, to perform surgical

---

[2]Intuitive Surgical acquires Computer Motion. Deal date: June 1, 2003/Deal #200310045, www.elsevierbi.com/deals/200310045

[3]www.intuitivesurgical.com

procedures that (a) require high levels of precision and (b) improve on the aforementioned and additional areas, has been seen in the utilization of robotic surgical systems (Patel, 2008). Furthermore, Drasin, Dutson, and Gracia (2004) have experimentally (through the use of the ZEUS® robotic system) concluded that the use of robotic assistance in advanced laparoscopic procedures and surgery is feasible and safe. Allen et al. (2010) consider shorter hospitalization time, smaller scars, and quicker healing to be highly advantageous for patients.

Historically, surgical robots were first introduced in 1987 with the first laparoscopic surgery, that is, a cholecystecotomy. PUMA 560 was the first nonlaparascopic robot used in robotic surgery in 1985. PROBOT further introduced a transurethral resecting surgery using PUMA 560. Later, ROBODOC[4,5] was developed by Integrated Surgical Systems of Sacramento, California. It was designed to move the femur to the correct position during hip replacement surgeries. Computer Motion developed the AESOP® Endoscope Positioner, a voice-activated robotic system for endoscopic surgery. In 1993, this became the first robot approved by the FDA for surgery. The HERMES® Control Center was also developed by Computer Motion and brought a centralized voice command and recognition system to the robotic medical devices. Integrated Surgical Systems (now Intuitive Surgical Inc.) redesigned the SRI Green Telepresence Surgery system and created the da Vinci® Surgical System, classified as a master–slave surgical system. It uses true 3D visualization and EndoWrist® actuation. It was approved by the FDA in July 2000 for general laparoscopic surgery and in November 2002 for mitral valve repair surgery and is also presently involved in a cardiac clinical trial in the United States for totally endoscopic CABG surgery. In 2001, the SOCRATES™ Robotic Telecollaboration System was created by Computer Motion. It included integrated telecommunication equipment along with robotic devices in order to provide remote surgical telecollaboration. This system was used for the first-ever transatlantic telesurgery performed (Butner and Ghodoussi, 2003). Computer Motion merged with Intuitive Surgical in June 2003. Recent advents in technology have resulted in new discoveries and improvements in endoscopic techniques, video imaging, and surgical instruments, which have enabled performing of a number

[4]http://en.wikipedia.org/wiki/Robotic_surgery

[5]ROBODOC: Surgical Robot Success Story. Retrieved 25 June 2013.

of traditionally manual surgeries through robotic surgery. With these advents, large incisions have been substituted by small ones, through which endoscopic cameras and robotic end effectors are inserted. These incisions (three to five of them in a typical robotic surgery) generally measure 1–5 mm in diameter. Therefore, surgeons are capable of performing surgeries without directly being in contact with the targeted tissues or organs. The robotic end effectors are equipped with limited haptic, optical, and force feedback sensors, which continuously transfer information to the surgeon. Image-processing equipment provides the surgeon with a realistic representation of the surgical scene with depth perception. The biggest achievement of this method is the level of detail that cannot be obtained by bare eyes.

Two different types of robot-aided surgery have emerged as practices, surgery utilizing robotic telescopic assistance through systems such as AESOP® and robotic procedural laparoscopy through implementation of systems such as da Vinci® or ZEUS® (Shew, Ostlie, and Holcomb, 2003). The former practice is semiautomated rather than fully automated due to a number of surgical tasks, for example, adjustments to robotic arms or optical fiber endoscopic cameras, requiring manual action. The latter practice, on the other hand, involves fully automated steps that involve control of robotic arms and instrumentation by the surgeon, who situates himself/herself in a special console typically located outside the sterilized area. Visual information on the surgical scene is conveyed from aforementioned sensors to special displays (occasionally binocular) to facilitate the surgeon's work.

Various types of robotic surgery have successfully been conducted on humans, namely, in urology (especially cystectomy) (Haber, Crouzet, and Gill, 2008); prostatectomy (White et al., 2010); nephrectomy (Patel, Menon, and Rogers, 2010); pediatric urology (Olsen, 2006); gynecology, more particularly trachelectromy (Al-Niaimi et al., 2011); myomectomy (Mao et al., 2007); gastrointestinal surgery with rectopexy (Munz et al., 2004); neurosurgery (Chan et al., 2009); hemicolectomy, cholecystectomy, different types of bypass, and adrenalectomy (Bochkarev, Ringley, and Oleynikov, 2005); neck surgery, particularly thymectomy (Castle and Kernstine, 2008); and vascular surgery (Martinez and Wiegand, 2004), providing great help to surgeons, considering the level of complexity that these surgeries exhibit, particularly when performed manually.

Applications in other fields, such as ophthalmology, have been attempted on porcine models (with the da Vinci® robotic system) (Tsui et al., 2010). Related to semiautomated robots, Mitchell et al. (2007) discuss the use of a steady arm, which is directly controlled by the surgeon and serves as a filter for hand tremor.

Robotic systems that are operated at a distance mainly consist of two entities, a robotic system and a surgeon station, from which the surgeon conducts the surgical procedure through controlling the robotic arms' movements via telemanipulation. This latter system is more technically known as a master–slave robotic system, where the surgeon is the master of the surgery in that he/she controls and supervises movements of the slave robotic arms and instruments from outside the sterile area of the surgical room. Advantages of such a master–slave robotic system for the surgeon include a comfortable body posture, intuitive instrument control, downscaled or upscaled instrument movements, hand tremor filtering, etc. (Meenink et al., 2010).

Inventors have pushed the advents and achievements in robotic surgery forward through their patented versions of such systems, with special focus on improving maneuverability/dexterity. US Patent No. 8170717 by Sutherland et al. (2012) is an example of this. In their invention, Sutherland et al. claim benefits of a magnetic resonance imaging (MRI) environment that, in combination with a microscope, performs neurosurgery. This system produces 16 degrees of freedom for the manipulation of 2 robotic arms.

Despite some drawbacks, surgical robots are becoming more of a necessity due to the advantages they hold over manual surgery. Their application has been proposed in remote distances on Earth as well as in space missions (Haidegger and Benyo, 2008), a practice that would allow surgeons to perform surgery from Earth on astronauts located aboard spaceships. Therefore, the most promising field for the future is teleoperation, through which surgeons are capable of performing surgery from a distance. Applying surgical robotic systems and their accompanying methods can result in minimal surgical invasion of patients' bodies, shorter hospitalization time, more accuracy, and convenience. The introduction of highly dexterous robots has enabled performing surgery at the micro level, which is difficult to achieve without the aid of advanced technology in imaging and robotic instrumentation. Horgan and Vanuno (2001) released a technical report on robotic systems in laparoscopic surgery. According to their experimental results, robotic surgery can provide a safe and effective alternative to conventional laparoscopic surgery. For thorough information regarding the use of robots in medicine, Taylor and Stoianovici's study (2003) provides a good summary of systems developed in time. Ma and Berkelman (2007) propose a compact laparoscopic surgical system. They put the results obtained from their compact system to test and compared them to the results they retrieved from manual surgery. The conclusion of their study suggests greater time efficiency and instrument manipulation through the use of their system. Figure 1.1 depicts a compact surgical system by Ma and Berkelman (2007).

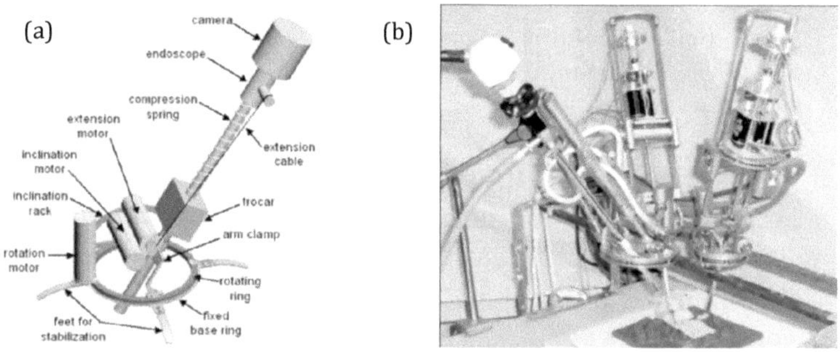


**Figure 1.1** Compact laparoscopic surgical system by Ma and Berkelman (2007). (a) Arm components and (b) arms in practice.

Lum et al. (2008) dispense a pilot study on the RAVEN surgical robot (Fig. 1.2). In their publication, they analyze the effect of time delay on the error rate of surgery during teleoperation.

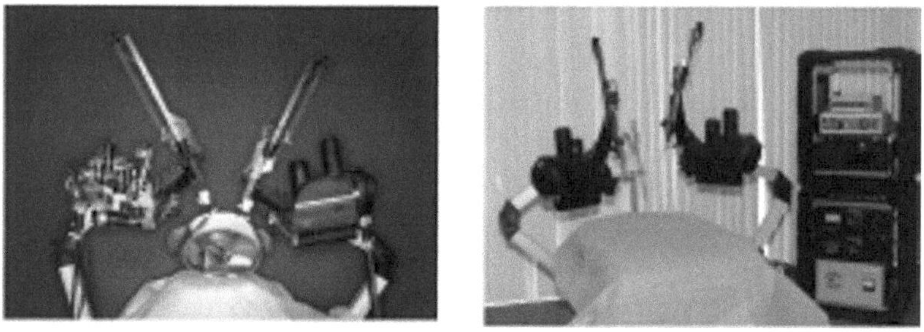

**Figure 1.2** The RAVEN surgical robot. (a) SolidWorks models and (b) arms in practice.

Mirbagheri et al. (2011) designed and developed a robotic system to handle the camera during laparoscopic surgeries, which is illustrated in Fig. 1.3.

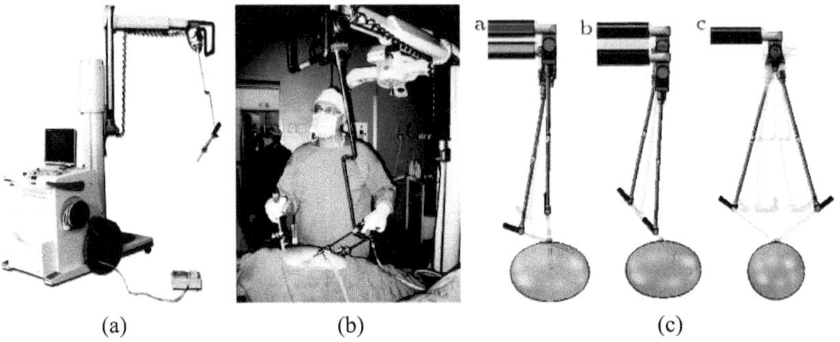


**Figure 1.3** The robotic cameraman by Mirbagheri et al. (2011). (a) The robotic cameraman, (b) the cameraman in use, and (c) dexterity and workspace.

For further information, refer to a collective review by Bann et al. (2003), entitled "Robotics in Surgery" and "Robotics in Surgery," published in *The Journal of Current Problems in Surgery* (2004). Robotic surgery is a field that will continue to draw attention. Hence, it constitutes the essence of this book.

## 1.3 Robotic Systems in Human Surgery

### 1.3.1 Surgical Robotic Systems and Their Advantages

As mentioned in the preceding descriptions, there are generally two types of robot-assisted surgery under use, one that utilizes robotic telescopic assistance, a group represented by systems such as AESOP®, and robotic procedural surgery, which is represented by systems such as da Vinci® and ZEUS®. Current robotic systems chiefly relate to and are used in conjunction with endoscopic techniques. In special cases, such as when using the SurgiScope system, these are used in conjunction with microscopic and electromyography (EMG) techniques. Other noncommercial surgical systems have been developed and tested that serve as hand stabilizers (tremor minimizers), rather than robots as distinct entities. Despite the level of automation, current surgical robotic systems are composed of four main entities: a surgical interface device or system, a computer controller, a number of robotic manipulator arms/instruments, and an imaging system. The lower the level of automation, the smaller the distinction among these entities, for example, the steady arm developed by Mitchell et al. (2007). The highest level of automation has been reached in teleoperation, where there is virtually no limitation in the potential distance between surgeon and patient. In these cases, there is no direct contact of the surgeon with robotic instruments; instead, the surgeon performs surgery from an interface device (usually enclosed in a console that comfortably houses the surgeon) by exerting a small amount of force on joysticks. These movements are conveyed to a computer controller, which processes them and instructs the robotic arms to follow the surgeon's movements, applied with a certain conversion factor, which are positioned on or near the operating table. Current surgical robotic arm systems are able to move with multiple degrees of freedom, simulating the movement of the human arm, elbow, and wrist.

Of substantial value for surgical robotic systems are the sensors they are equipped with. Recent trends include equipping robotic arm end effectors with limited haptic, force feedback, and optical sensors in order to achieve optimal visualization of the surgical scene as the surgery proceeds. Information retrieved from the sensors is transferred to the computer controllers and from there to monitors, where the vision quality and level of detail render this procedure superior to unaided vision for surgeons. Leading companies in robotic surgery offer high-resolution, 3D equipment for a highly precise perception of the surgical scene, allowing surgeons to accurately perceive the depth and distance of organs. The benefits of using a robotic system to perform surgery on patients will be described herein and include:

- *The ability to perform surgery from a remote location.* In the case of teleoperation, it is possible to operate on a patient from a distance, including cases when the patient is in outer space. Therefore, convenience is one of the reasons why this field has received attention and investment. With recent achievements in the field of robotics, surgeons no longer need to be directly in touch with patients' tissues or surgical instrumentation, nor must they directly observe the ongoing surgical scene (with bare eyes). Instead, every aspect of the surgery is performed from a special console located outside the sterile zone. This applies to occasions where both the patient and the surgeon are in the same room or building, as well as remote battlefields or when the patient is in space. The potential applications are virtually endless, all due to the ability to operate independently from a great distance.

- *Minimal incision on the patient's body.* Laparoscopic techniques are well known in the field of robotic surgery. Recent robotic systems claim the benefits of minimally invasive practices to access damaged tissue during surgery. Typically, three to five small openings are made around the area of interest on the patient's body, and robotic instruments and cameras are inserted therein. These practices allow for less trauma, quicker recovery, and shorter hospitalization time.
- *Enhanced visibility and information access.* Despite each case demanding different levels of visual detail, there is a natural need for reasonable visibility during surgery. In theory, the better the virtual information obtained from sensors, the more successful and precise the resulting surgical procedure. Modern robotic surgical systems are equipped with large-sized, high-magnification monitors that continuously display the surgical scene. Due to combinations in sensors of the latest technology, the surgeon has access to a large variety of parameters related to the surgical procedure: parameters that help him/her perform a more successful intervention. In some cases, 3D technology is incorporated into the system in order to provide the best possible visual guidance to the surgeon. All the information described in this section considers the fact that robotic systems used in surgery employ endoscopic techniques; therefore, it is important that these breakthroughs be considered in the appropriate context.
- *Hand movement scaling and tremor cancellation.* In robotic surgery, two major changes to direct surgeon hand movements are filtering and scaling. Filtering generates very precise movements of robotic instruments, which eventually minimizes trauma to patients' surgical wounds. In cases when endoscopic techniques are employed in surgery, filtering becomes a necessity due to hand tremor being leveraged and

magnified at the tip of the instrument. Regarding movement scaling, some types of surgery involve instrument movements that are very small in scale, sometimes so small that they are almost impossible to accomplish with bare hands. Therefore, downscaling a surgeon's hand movements on the joystick through digital processing in the main computer controller enables surgery at the micro level. Motion scaling also facilitates ambidexterity. The level of scaling on surgeons' hand movements can in fact be tuned both up and down.
Prasad et al. (2004) designed a study to compare the surgical accuracy between conventional laparascopic instruments and a robotic surgical system (ZEUS®) and evaluate the importance of tremor filtration and motion scaling in robotic systems. They concluded that the enhanced accuracy seen in robotic surgical systems mainly results from motion scaling rather than tremor filtration. Cassilly et al. published a journal paper in 2004 entitled "Optimizing Motion Scaling and Magnification in Robotic Surgery." They concluded that motion scaling can reduce the number of errors at higher magnification. However, it can also increase the task completion time by a great amount. Thus, optimization of both the motion scaling and magnification components of robotic systems to balance precision and speed seems necessary (Cassilly et al., 2004).

- *High dexterity*. Naturally, six degrees of freedom suffice in determining and reaching a certain point in space. These degrees of freedom include the *x-y-z* direction of movement toward the point of interest, as well as rotation in each direction. Standard laparoscopic equipment typically offers four degrees of freedom and is both tiresome and limited in mobility. The latest robotic systems provide anywhere from 7 to 18 degrees of freedom. A simple reasoning lies behind this rationale. Although systems with six degrees of freedom suffice in reaching any point in space, they do not account for different configurations and trajectories that may be necessary to overcome obstacles. If we consider throat surgery, it is not possible to conduct surgery with six degrees of freedom, due to any instrumentation needing to take a configuration compatible with the shape of the throat. Therefore, multiple degrees of freedom are not an option; they are a necessity due to the complexity of human anatomy.

- *Consistent results*. During manual surgery, any sudden movements or impulses by the surgeon can result in grave consequences. Furthermore, the success of manual surgery largely depends on factors such as the surgeon's ability, experience, and, especially, the length of the surgery: fatigue certainly affects performance, especially by increasing risk of accidents. However, when operating with a surgical robot, a comfortable seat is provided to the surgeon, and a robot cannot experience fatigue over the course of a surgery. Unless a fatal error occurs with the computer-controlling system (which is very unlikely and would, in any case, be amortized by safety systems), there is virtually no risk of major damage to the patient's tissue. In this aspect, robotic surgery is superior to manual surgery.
- *Comfortable posture for the surgeon*. The success of manual surgery generally depends on the surgeon's capabilities and experience and the length of the surgery. Through utilization of robotic surgical systems, the surgeon sits in an ergonomically designed surgeon's console and operates with more confidence and greater maneuverability. The surgeon's performance is also less affected by fatigue due to the length of surgery.
- *Education and training*. Results have suggested a strong positive correlation between the surgeons' training and robotic surgery success. Apparently, there is a learning curve for every new robotic system that is introduced to the medical community. Before conducting robotic surgery on a human being, a surgeon undergoes a long process of training that involves a certain number of tests on porcine or animal subjects. After a threshold number of test surgeries is performed (specific for each type of surgical procedure and/or robotic system), it can be determined whether the newly trained surgeon is ready to perform surgery on humans. Bann et al. (2003) have extensively analyzed different aspects of learning curves and trends related to the training of surgeons in conducting robotic surgery. Prasad et al. (2002) also discuss skill improvement in correlation with increases in

the number of preliminary tests performed on nonhuman models. The bottom line is that training is crucial: with more tests, surgeons' skills sequentially improve, thereby ensuring their readiness for human surgery.

To conclude, robotic surgery exhibits improved features as compared to manual or lowly automated surgery. Enhanced dexterity, high precision, consistency of results, long-distance operation, minimal incision, and enhanced visibility define typical robotic surgery. With such properties, there is certainly a bright future for this field of medicine.

## 1.3.2 Applications of Robotics in Surgery

### 1.3.2.1 Neurosurgery

The first application of robotics in neurosurgery was enabling a stereotactic biopsy (Kwoh et al., 1988). The first robot developed for such applications was PUMA 560, as mentioned before (Fig. 1.4). On the other side, the Swiss Minerva system was developed for high-precision needle placement, while working in conjunction with a computed tomography (CT) scanner and providing five degrees of freedom (Fankhauser et al., 1994).

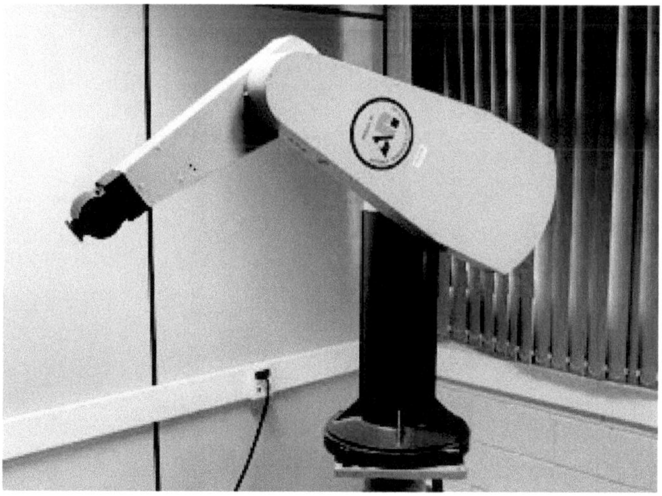

**Figure 1.4** The PUMA 560 robot was first used in neurosurgery [Kwoh et al., 1988].

Another robotic system developed in Italy included a Stabuli Rx 90 robot, a microscope controller and imaging equipment. It has already been successfully tested (Giorgi et al., 2000). A similar technique is utilized by the SurgiScope$^{TM}$ robotic system (Fig. 1.5), which employs microscopic techniques and an MRI scanner to first generate a map of the brain. The surgeon then plots the course of the surgery on the computer system, and eventually the robot delivers/operates on the brain with extreme precision. NeuroMate$^{TM}$ was developed by Integrated Surgical Systems (Davis, CA) and consists of an image-guided robotic system for stereotactic functional brain surgery (Fig. 1.6). It includes a presurgical planning imagery workstation, which consists of a planning device that serves as a plotter for the subsequent surgery. By first acquiring brain map data, the surgeon can determine the course of the surgery and convey it successfully. For a comprehensive review of neurosurgery equipment and technology, and how robots are assisting this field (Alexander and Maciunas, 1999).

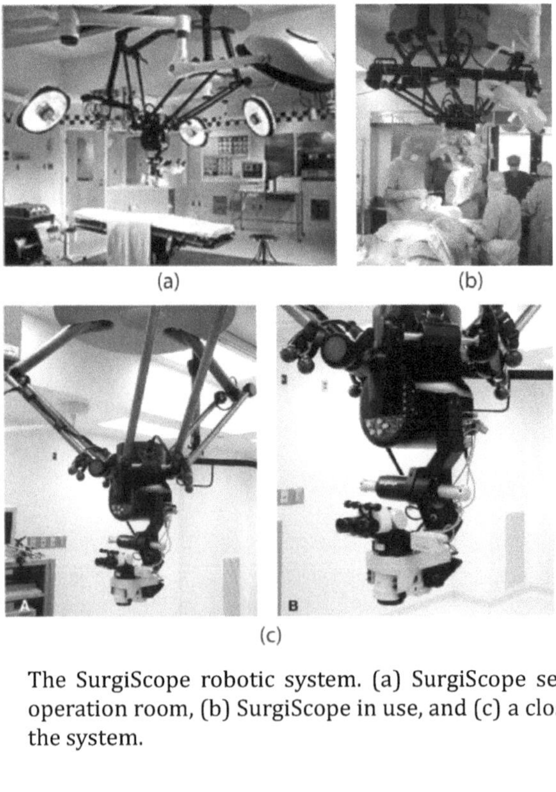


**Figure 1.5** The SurgiScope robotic system. (a) SurgiScope set up in an operation room, (b) SurgiScope in use, and (c) a closer view of the system.

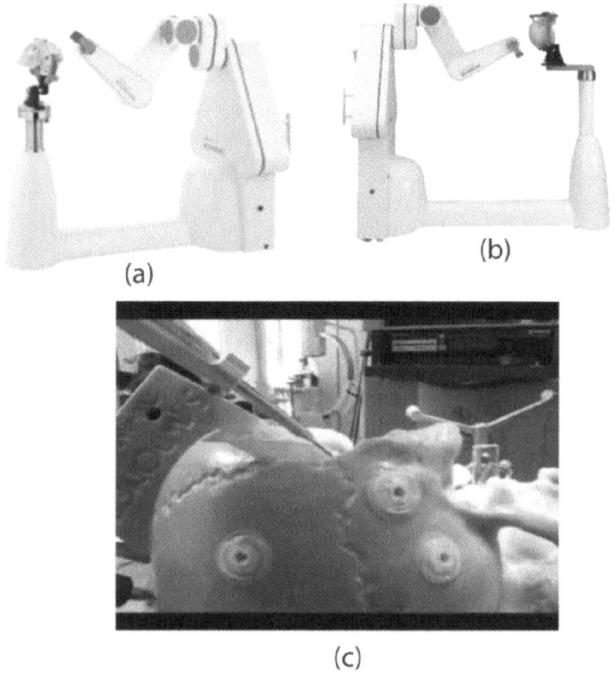


**Figure 1.6** The NueroMate robotic surgical system. (a) A left-side view, (b) a right-side view, and (c) a closer view in operation mode.

#### 1.3.2.2 Orthopedic applications

- *Hip replacement.* The best representative robotic system is called ROBODOC (by Integrated Surgical Systems), which is composed of three elements: a planning station, a cutting robot, and a control panel. ROBODOC (Fig. 1.7) was invented by Howard Paul, DVM, and William Bargar, MD, and delivers five degrees of freedom.[6] A typical hip replacement procedure involves placement of three locator pins in the hip that define anatomic features of the patient. A full CT scan follows this. The surgeon then plans the schedule for the insertion of the implant, which is conveyed to the control system of ROBODOC. The robot then precisely mills the part to be replaced, continuously monitored by the surgeon. Eventually the implant is installed through manual methods.

[6]http://www.robodoc.com/eng/orthodoc.html

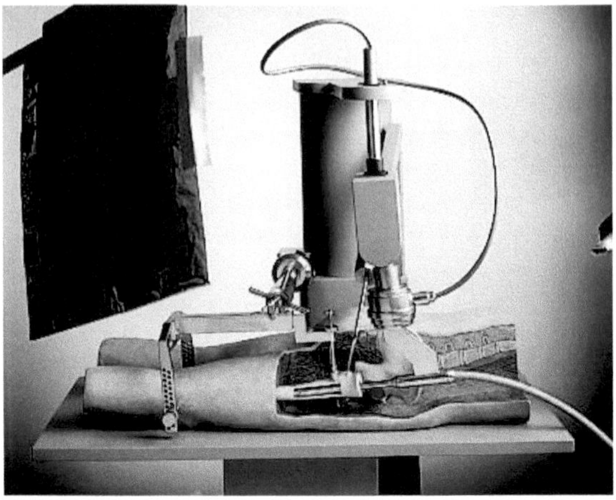

**Figure 1.7** The ROBODOC surgical system.

- *Knee replacement.* It is crucial that the prosthesis and limb be precisely aligned, which is why robotic surgery seems like an optimal alternative. By using robotic assistance, it is also possible to machine the surface of bones in direct contact with the prosthesis in order to improve the match between the two. B. L. Davies in London developed ACROBOT (Fig. 1.8), precisely for knee replacement surgery (Jakopec et al., 2001). ACROBOT uses a force-controlled lever, directly operated by the surgeon, to perform surgery.

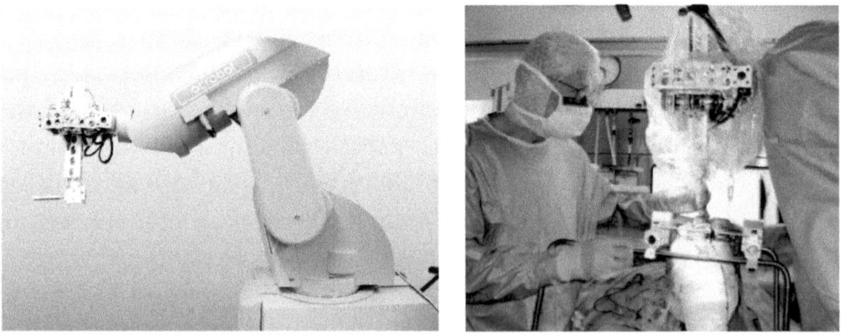

(a) (b)

**Figure 1.8** The ACROBOT surgical system for knee replacement. (a) A side view of the system and (b) ACROBOT in use.

The robot features a rotary cutter that can cut various shapes in order to facilitate implantation. A control system prevents the surgeon from excessively moving the cutter. Typically, both the femur and the tibia are held firmly against the surgical bed to prevent unwanted movement during the course of the surgery.

After the computer takes CT images and the surgeon chooses the prosthesis, he/she then chooses 20 to 30 points on the exposed bone surface and initiates cutting of the bone. Eventually the patella is prepared manually, and the prosthesis is placed in the same fashion. Another robotic system worth mentioning is called Computer-Assisted Surgical Robotics (CASPAR) (Fig. 1.9), which is a computer-based planning system used in autonomous implantation of knee prostheses. The featured computer permits virtual implantation of a prosthesis. The robot system subsequently performs the intervention. The Compact Robot System for Image-Guided Orthopedic Surgery (CRIGOS) also follows a similar process of operation (Brandt et al., 2000).

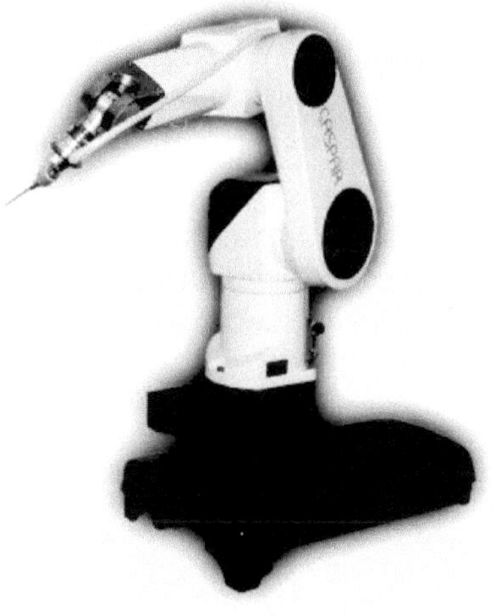

**Figure 1.9** The CASPAR robotic surgical system.

### 1.3.2.3 Urology applications

A seven-degrees-of-freedom robot was first used in 1989 for transurethral resection of the prostate (TURP) in London (Davies et al., 1989). This system, however, did not succeed in the market due to the development of better techniques. Trials to develop a good robotic system continued through the 1990s, when some "urobots" emerged that featured online imaging and 3D prostate model simulation, a computer-controlled system, and a rectoscope mounted on a robotic arm. The robot initially measured the prostate, and then an ultrasound probe performed scans to build a 3D representation of the prostate. The surgeon used the model to plot the cut of the cavity. Eventually the robot, monitored by the surgeon, performed the prostatectomy by cutting cones.

The best results in urology have been achieved with the introduction of the da Vinci® surgical robot (Fig. 1.10). More specifically, robot-assisted anatomic radical prostatectomy (RARP) is one of the techniques that have received the highest level of attention. Typically, this technique involves making six openings: one 12 mm opening near the umbilicus for the binocular scope, two 8 mm openings on the left side of the patient for the robotic arms, another 5 mm opening on the left to be used by the surgical assistant, while both a 10 mm and a 5 mm opening are placed on the right for retraction, suction, and insertion of sutures. Initially, lymphadenectomy is performed and then the seminal vesicles are dissected. Subsequently, the bladder and prostate are mobilized and the prostatic apex and fascia are exposed. The bladder neck is transected afterward, and the pedicles are exposed to allow the dissection of nerves. Then the puborectalis muscle is dissected from the urethra, while the latter is cut anteriorly and posteriorly to allow cutting of the rectourethralis muscle. The specimen is installed in the retrieval bag, followed by the formation of the urethrovesicular anastomosis. Eventually the specimen is removed and the incisions are closed (Tewari et al., 2002).

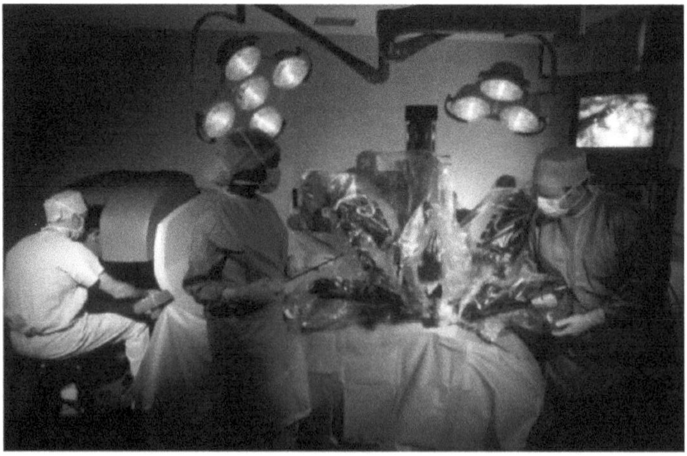

**Figure 1.10** The da Vinci® robotic surgical system.

Robotic surgical systems have been utilized in prostate biopsies and to obtain percutaneous access to the kidney (PAKY; Fig. 1.11) (Cadeddu et al., 1997). Kidney biopsies have been achieved through coupling robotic arms with image-capturing devices, for example, CT and a computer system. The Remote Center of Motion (RCM) is a robotic system that uses such a combination and has successfully been tested in long-distance surgery, with patients in Milano, Italy, and the surgeon conducting surgery from Baltimore, Maryland (Micali et al., 2000). Therefore, robotic PAKY has proven to be feasible, safe, and effective. A robot-assisted nephrectomy was achieved in 2001 with the use of the ZEUS® robotic system (Guillonneau et al., 2001), while a kidney transplant was successfully performed with the da Vinci® system one year later (Hoznek et al., 2002).

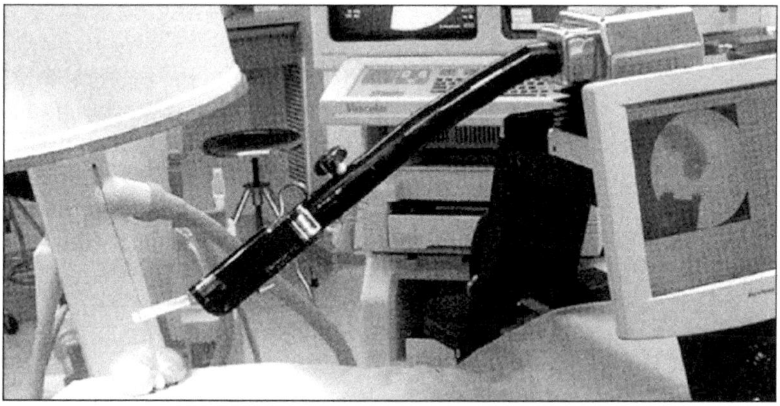

**Figure 1.11** The PAKY surgical robot.

The Probot (Fig. 1.12) is a robotic system that has been used in TURP (Ng et al., 1993). The original robotic arm was adapted through the addition of a transurethral ultrasonographic probe that directly measured the gland size at the beginning of the procedure for simulation of a 3D model, which permits the surgeon to select parts to be removed by the diathermic cutter. The Robotic System for Biopsy and Interventional Therapy of Mammary Lesions (ROBITOM) represents a versatile robot for low-force procedures. It is used in breast lesion diagnosis and biopsy simultaneously (Kaiser et al., 2000).

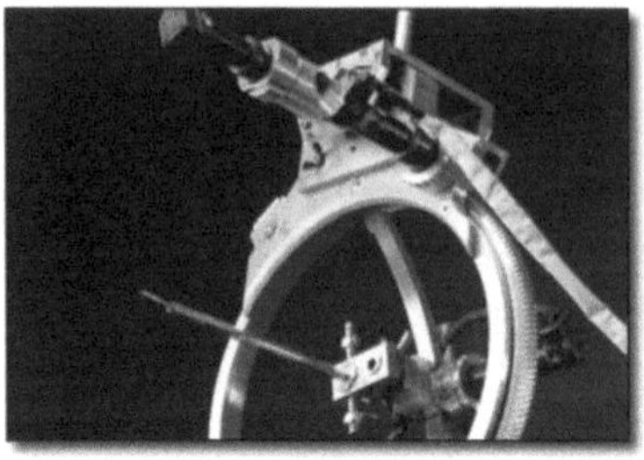

(a)

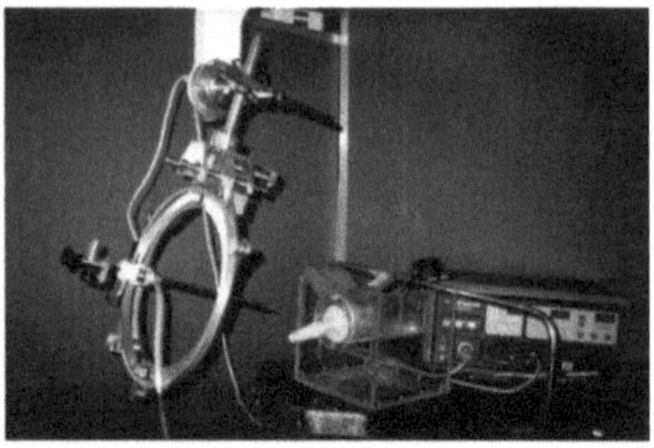

(b)

**Figure 1.12** The Probot surgical system. (a) A detailed view and (b) a general view.

#### 1.3.2.4 Cardiovascular surgery applications

- *Vascular surgery applications.* In the vascular field, the adoption of laparoscopic techniques has proceeded slowly because of the high level of complexity and the limited dexterity that laparoscopic techniques provide. With the introduction of robotic systems, this field of surgery has the potential to develop fast (Fig. 1.13).

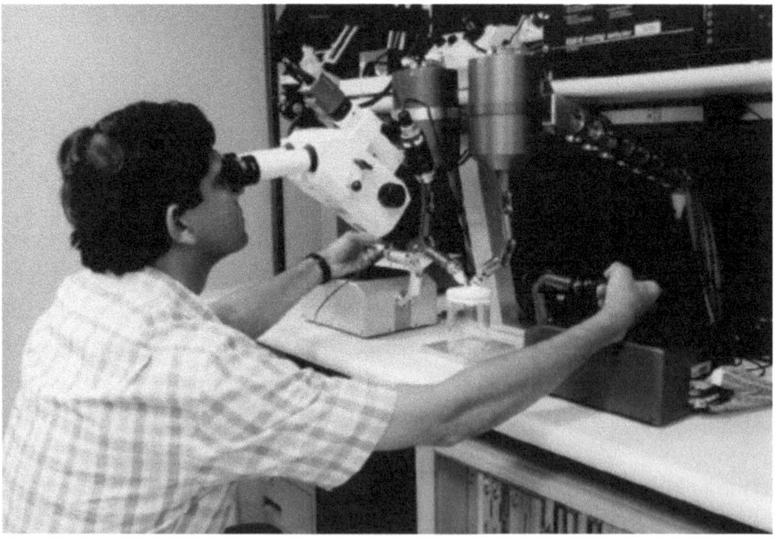

**Figure 1.13** Robot-assisted microsurgery (RAMS).

A first trial in carotid arteriotomy on mice in 2001 (by Le Roux, using the robot-assisted microsurgery [RAMS] microdexterity enhancement system) was successful, though the overall procedure lasted three times longer than manual surgery (Le Roux et al., 2001). One year later, Wisselink et al. (2002) tested the feasibility of constructing aortobifemoral bypass grafts with the aid of the ZEUS® robotic system.

- *Cardiac surgery applications.* Cardiac surgery boasts the publication of extensive robotic literature. Robot-aided techniques have permitted surgeons to more effectively conduct complex procedures that have previously been performed through a median sternotomy.
  - CABG. Extensive experience has been collected through the introduction of robotics in CABG. The main robotic systems utilized in this procedure worldwide are the ZEUS® and da Vinci® robotic systems. Judging from this extensive experience from clinics around the world, robotic systems are fully capable of performing CABG. Surgeons continue to become more skillful in using the available robotic systems, which will continuously improve the safety and efficiency of CABG in the future. Currently, fully endoscopic CABG is performed on patients with limited coronary artery disease. The wide use of this method necessitates development of methods that facilitate anastomosis.
  - Mitral valve surgery. The first trials in this field involved the use of the Heartport (Redwood City, CA) procedure, which enabled the use of smaller incisions than the traditional sternotomy, although visibility was of low quality. Onnasch in Leipzig, Germany, has achieved the greatest results in mitral valve surgery. Generally, his team employs AESOP 3000® (Fig. 1.14) to perform this surgical procedure; however, they have experimented with combining AESOP® and the da Vinci® robotic system to conclude the procedure (Onnasch et al., 2002). In general, these trials suggest that mitral valve surgery with robot-aided techniques is feasible. However, success here is strongly related to the ease of the learning curve.

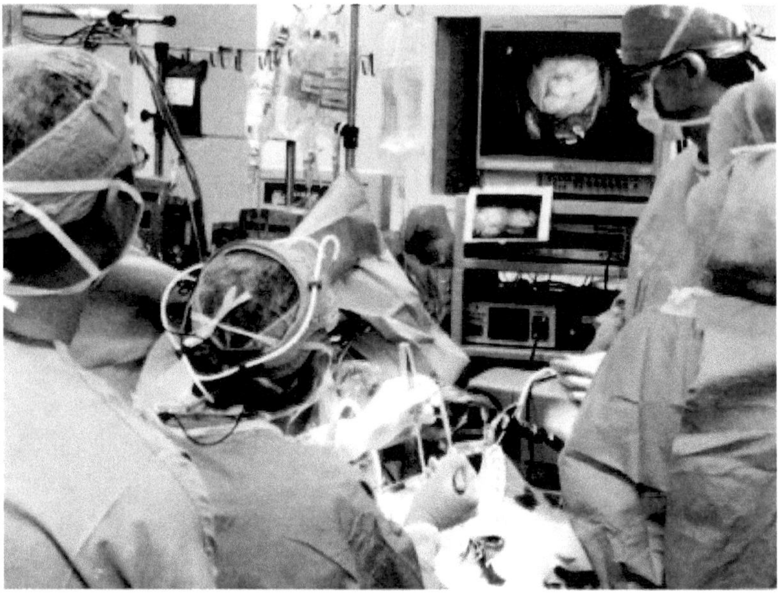

**Figure 1.14** Robotic mitral valve surgery via AESOP®.[7]

Kypson, Nifong, and Chitwood (2003) also conclude that the use of robotic systems is beneficial in performing mitral valve surgery since they provide high dexterity to operate in tight spaces and allow for ambidextrous suture placement (Figs. 1.15 and 1.16).

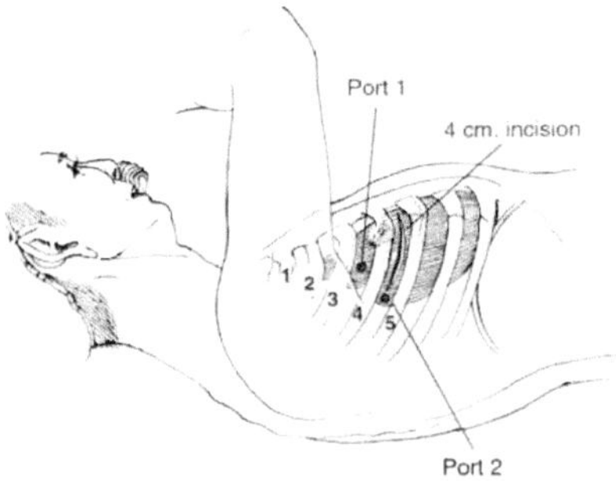


**Figure 1.15** Proper patient position for robotic mitral valve surgery by Kypson, Nifong, and Chitwood (2003).

---

[7]http://www.womensheart.org/content/Newsletter/ArchivedArticles/2001_06_article_MVSurgeryWithAesopRobot.asp

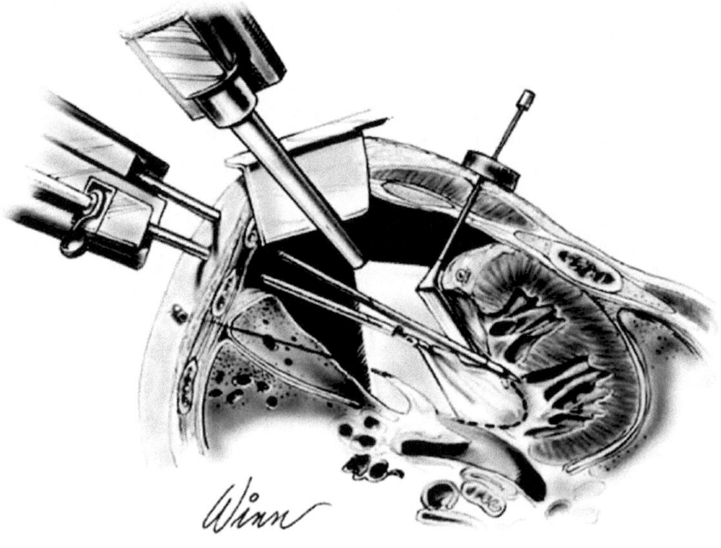


**Figure 1.16** Cross section of the operative site in mitral valve surgery by Kypson, Nifong, and Chitwood (2003).

Siwek and Reynolds (2007) illustrate the steps and techniques of robotic mitral valve repair in their article.

- Atrial septal surgery. The da Vinci® Surgical System has been used by Torraca et al. (2002) in Milano, Italy, in repairing atrial septal defects (ASDs), as well as by Argenziano et al. (2002). Their results again suggest the success of robot-aided methods in delivering this type of surgery.

#### 1.3.2.5 Gynecology applications

Robot-aided technology and methods have found application in gynecology as well. The ZEUS® and da Vinci® systems have been used successfully in some types of gynecologic surgery. For instance, Margossian et al. (1998) have extensively tested these two robotic systems in microsurgical anastomoses. Degueldre et al. in 2000 treated tubal reanastomoses with the da Vinci® system in Belgium. Despite concluding that such procedures are feasible and hold advantages such as enhanced visibility, the authors mentioned a lack of haptic feedback as problematic in a paper submitted on their related work (Degueldre et al., 2000). In 2002, the da Vinci® robot was implemented by a group at the University of Texas in laparoscopic hysterectomy and bilateral salpingo-oophorectomy (Diaz-Arrastia et al., 2002). To summarize, the authors concluded that their results suggest the superiority of robotic systems in gynecologic surgery as compared to standard laparoscopy. This is mostly due to robotic systems offering enhanced visualization, superior dexterity due to multiple degrees of freedom, and minimization of fatigue with the introduction of comfortable housing of the surgeon and easy-to-control joysticks. The authors see potential improvements in the development of intrapelvic instruments, such as Babcock clamps, harmonic scalpels, and bipolar cautery. In 2011, Tchartchian et al. concluded that a dynamic laparoscope manipulator can facilitate convenient solo surgery, which mainly results from superior image stability and less extended intervention as a result of the camera correction as compared to conventional laparoscopy (Tchartchian et al., 2011).

#### 1.3.2.6 Ophthalmic surgery

Ocular surgery is another field where the benefits of surgical robotic systems can be exploited, though no specific care has been given to developing a dedicated commercial surgical system for this purpose. Studies report trials to perform eye surgery with the da Vinci® robot, which have achieved success to a certain extent. Thus, tests on extraocular surgery have been performed on porcine models, and the multiple degrees of freedom that the da Vinci® system features seem not to be of much value in this small-scale surgery. This is caused by the robotic instrumentation pivot point being external to the eye, which significantly decreases the dexterity of the robotic end effectors.

Furthermore, the robotic instrumentation is bulky. However, more attention is expected to be paid to robotic ophthalmic surgery in the future. Dalvand and Shirinzadeh (2013) studied the control of a parallel robot for use in minimally invasive surgery/microsurgery. This robot is shown in Fig. 1.17.

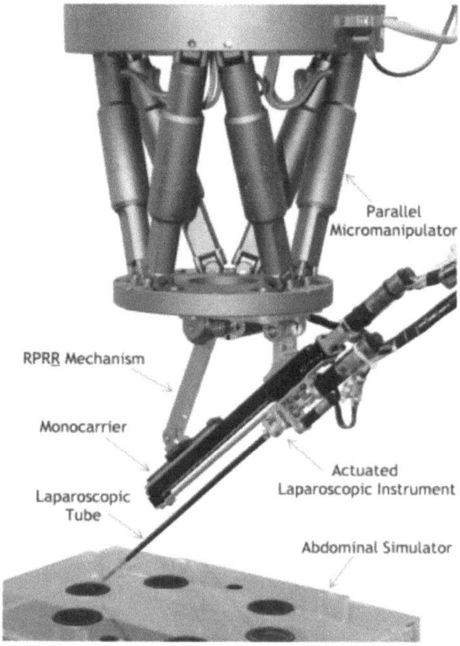


**Figure 1.17** The parallel robot for microsurgery by Dalvand and Shirinzadeh (2013).

#### 1.3.2.7 Hair transplant

Restoration Robotics Inc. has released a robot for hair transplants, called ARTAS® (Fig. 1.18). This robot provides the surgeon with more maneuverability and precision.

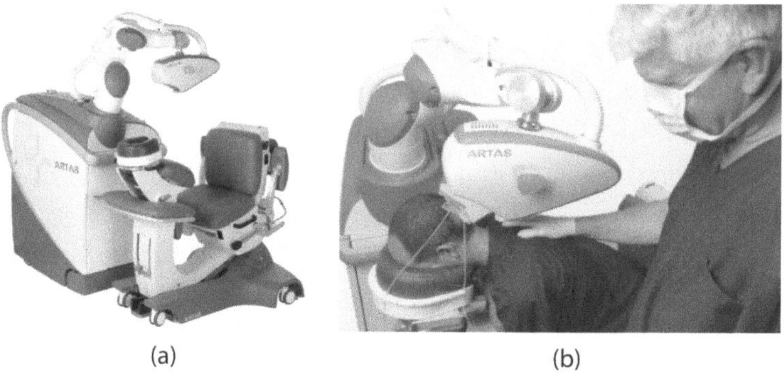


**Figure 1.18** The ARTAS robotic surgical system. (a) A general view and (b) ARTAS® in use.

### 1.3.2.8 Other applications

Abdominal techniques in robotic surgery have received less analysis and fewer reports than cardiac procedures. The implementation of robotic surgery in abdominal surgery clearly offers advantages that were discussed in the preceding paragraphs. When it comes to tremor cancelation, however, generally less emphasis is given when performing this type of surgery. Despite this fact, other benefits are important in distinguishing this method from regular laparoscopy.

- *Laparoscopic cholecystectomy.* The first report of a robotic laparoscopic cholecystectomy was submitted in 1998 in Belgium by Himpens, Leman, and Cadiere (1998). To perform surgery, the authors utilized the MONA™ system by Intuitive Surgical (Sunnydale, CA), the same company that developed the da Vinci® system. Marescaux et al. (2001) from Strasbourg, France, used the ZEUS® system to conduct this surgery. In both cases, robotic assistance was conclusively feasible, safe, and comparable in operative and recovery times with standard laparoscopic cholecystectomy.
- *Obesity surgery.* The MONA™ robotic system was the first to be used in an obesity surgical procedure (adjustable silicone gastric banding) by Cadeire et al. (1999) in Belgium. The procedure was successful and led to further experimentation and developments in the field.
- *Biliary surgery.* A report of 2001 determined the feasibility of repair of created common bile duct injury on a porcine model with the ZEUS® robotic system (Sweeney and Rattner, 2002). The report deemed this type of surgery possible, though the relatively high cost and procedure time were mentioned as obstacles in the widespread use of this method.

In 2008, David J. Terris and Shivan H. Amin talked about applications of robotics in neck surgery (Fig. 1.19). They believe that robots have a future in neck surgery if designed more specifically for this type of operation and accompanied with more customized instrumentation. Performing robotic neck surgery can significantly reduce operative times (David and Amin, 2008).

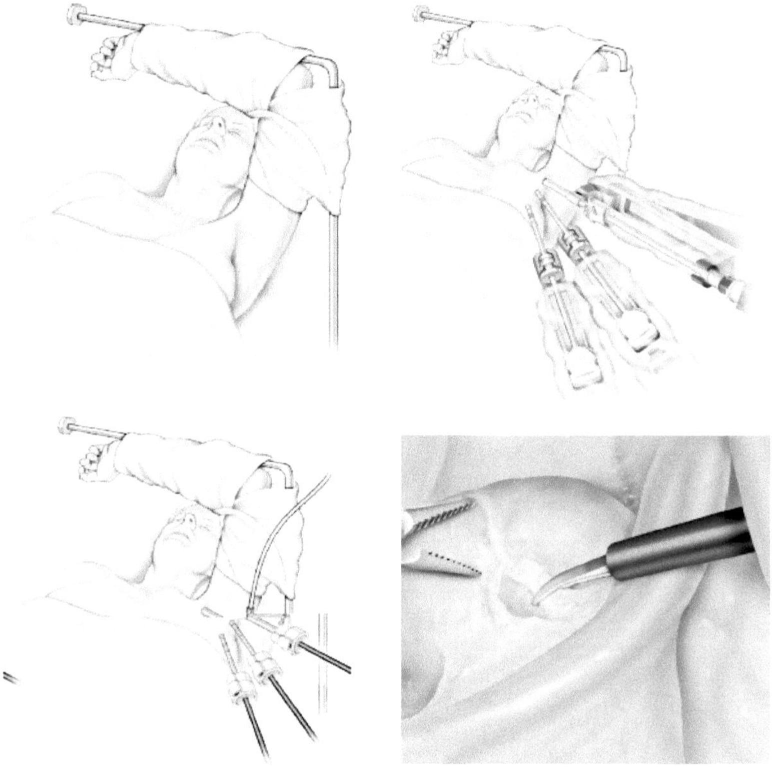

**Figure 1.19** Robotic neck surgery by Terris and Amin (2008).

Bochkarev, Ringley, and Oleynikov (2005) discuss robotic-assisted operative techniques in general surgery. Their article explains how to use a robotic surgical system to perform many types of surgeries. It also provides pictorial illustrations of various robotic-assisted operations, as can be seen in the following pictures (Fig. 1.20a–d).

Robotic surgery is an emerging field and is entering many different types of surgical operations. While current commercial robotic surgical systems are big and expensive, the future of robotic surgery is seen in small, special-purpose, lower-cost, and possibly disposable robots (Gomes, 2011).

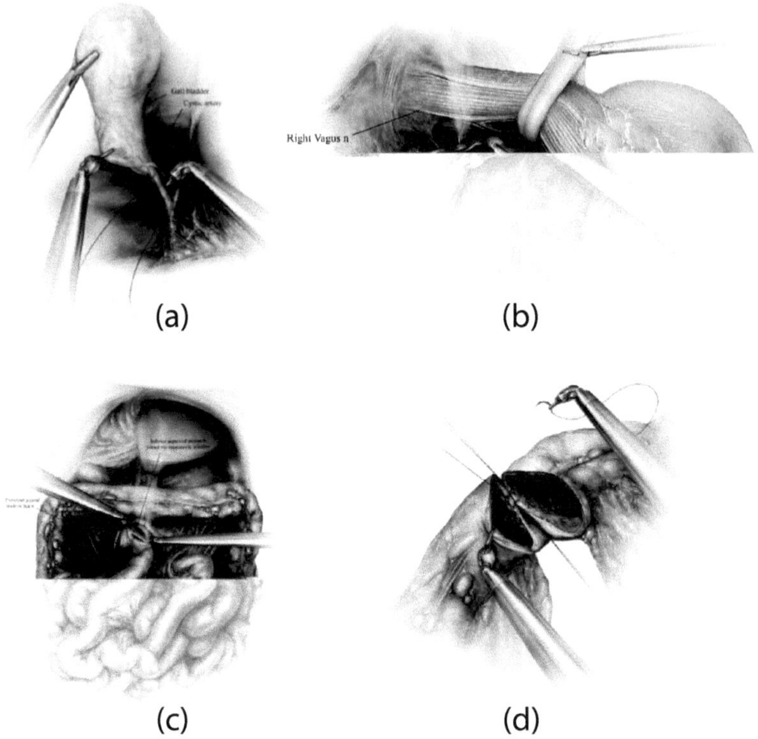


**Figure 1.20** Operative techniques in robotic-assisted laparascopic (a) cholecystectomy, (b) Nissen fundoplication, (c) gastric bypass, and (d) left hemicolectomy by Bochkarev, Ringley, and Oleynikov (2005).

## Problem Set

1. What did the first versions of robots mostly consist of?
2. Who first used "robotics" as a term?
3. Describe the three laws of robotics.
4. Define the term "robot".
5. What are different classes of robots?
6. What were the two major companies that pioneered the development and marketing of surgical robotic systems? What systems did they develop?
7. Describe robotic surgery.

8. What main entities does a robotic system consist of? Describe them.
9. What are patient-side benefits of robotic surgery?
10. What are surgeon-side benefits of robotic surgery?
11. What are the two different types of robot-aided surgery? Describe them.
12. Technically, what are the four entities current surgical robotic systems comprise? Describe them.
13. Name some surgeries robots have entered into.

# Chapter 2

# Surgical Robots' Kinematics and Workspace

## 2.1 Kinematics of Robotic Manipulators

### 2.1.1 Introduction to Kinematics of Robotic Manipulators

Kinematics is the study of the motion of objects without consideration of forces that generate the motion. Kinematics of robotic manipulators is the analysis of the movements and geometrical configurations and constraints of robotic structures during manipulation. It deals with geometrical properties of the robotic system and time derivatives of position variables such as velocity and acceleration.

In this chapter we start with a general description of robotic manipulators and continue with an introduction to the mathematical notation that is mostly used in the kinematic analysis of robots. Then some mathematical tools are further described as prerequisites to this knowledge, which assist us in finding out the kinematic attitude of one link with respect to an adjoining link in a robotic system. In other words, one can find out how two adjacent links move with respect to each other when position variables change. This eventually leads to derivation of the Denavit–Hartenberg (D–H)

*Robotic Surgery: Smart Materials, Robotic Structures, and Artificial Muscles*
Mohsen Shahinpoor and Siavash Gheshmi

ISBN 978-981-4316-23-1 (Hardcover), 978-981-4463-51-5 (eBook)
www.panstanford.com

homogeneous transformation. Both direct and inverse kinematics analyses of robotic manipulators are covered in this chapter, and some interesting robotic engineering problems are discussed.

### 2.1.2 General Description of Robotic Manipulators

A robotic manipulator is an open-loop chain of links connected in series by either prismatic or revolute joints. One end of the manipulator is attached to a supporting base and is stationary; the other end is relatively free and commonly attached to a specialized tool such as an endoscopic camera. The free end can reach out to different points of its workspace to perform a specific task. For instance, it can carry an electrode so that it welds two objects together, it can have a gripper to pick objects from one location and place them in another, and it can be facilitated with medical instruments like trocars, grippers, and suturing needles to perform surgical tasks robotically. The location and orientation of the free end is the result of the collective effect of translation and rotation of each joint of a robotic manipulator chain of links. Such motions are controlled by actuators that are electrical, magnetic, hydraulic, or pneumatic.

The central issue in industrial robotic manipulation is the ability to position the robotic free end at a specified location with a specified orientation at a given time, which is the core of flexible and automated manufacturing.

Figure 2.1 shows a standard six-axis robotic manipulator possessing a base (waist), shoulder, elbow, and wrist capable of pitch, roll, and yaw motions, as well as gripping motion. Mathematically, the position and orientation of the free end or the robotic end effector can be described in terms of the position and orientation of a coordinate frame attached to the end effector with respect to an inertial reference coordinate frame, which is usually fixed at the base of the robotic manipulator, as shown in Fig. 2.2.

The combination of the spatial location and orientation of the end effector (kinematic attitude) can be described mathematically by means of $4 \times 4$ homogeneous transformations. These homogeneous transformations are used to solve both the direct and the inverse kinematic problems of robotic manipulation.

Referring to Fig. 2.3, the direct kinematics problem in robotics is to find the kinematic attitude, given the vector of the joint displacements, $\theta_i = [\theta_1 \theta_2 \theta_3 \ldots \theta_n]^T$ for an $n$-axis robotic manipulator.

On the other hand, the inverse kinematics problem for robotic manipulators involves finding the vector of the joint displacements $\theta_i$, $i = 1, 2, \ldots, N$, for $n$-axis robotic manipulators, given the kinematic attitude of the gripper with respect to the base coordinates. Normally, the latter is the most desirable problem to solve because it is at the heart of flexible automated manufacturing operations and assembly processes. On the other hand, the direct kinematic solutions are used for special applications such as direct trajectory planning or obstacle collision prevention algorithms.

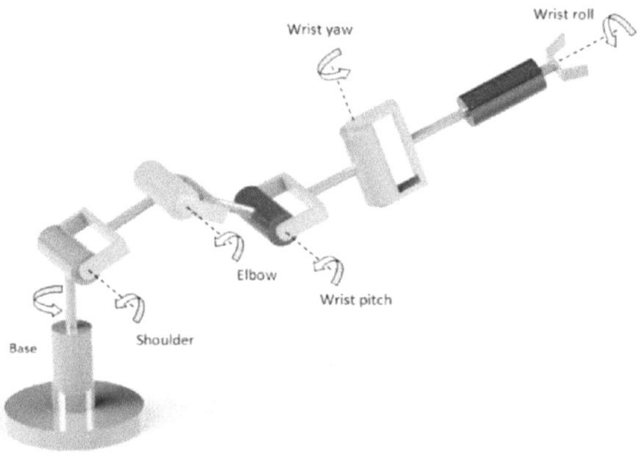


**Figure 2.1** Typical six-axis revolute robotic manipulator.

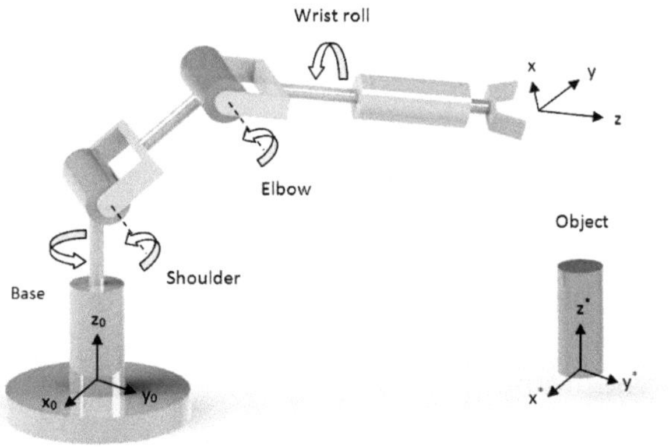


**Figure 2.2** Relative configuration of the gripper and base coordinate frame in a robotic manipulator.

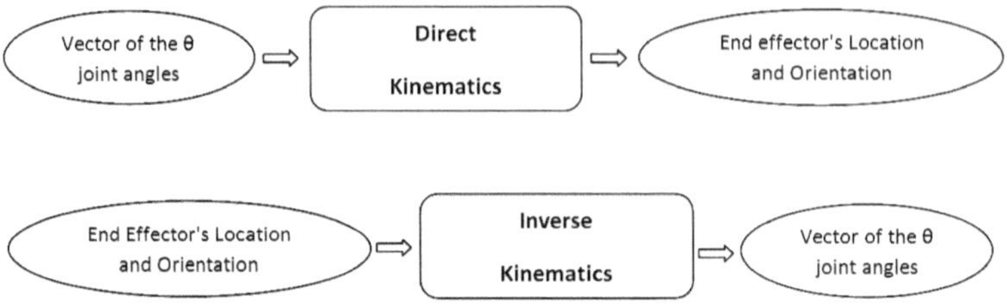


**Figure 2.3** Definition of direct and inverse kinematics.

In the following section, a brief description of the mathematical notation used throughout this text is described.

### 2.1.3 A Brief Description of Mathematical Notation

Conventional notation for the representation of vectors, scalars, and matrices are used throughout the text. In the following section you can find different notations used in the text:

- Presuperscripts denote descriptive information regarding coordinate frames. For instance, ${}^{A}\boldsymbol{r}$ is a position vector described with respect to frame **A**.
- Frame **A** itself is represented by a 4 × 4 homogenous transformation that describes the location of its origin and relative rotation with respect to a universal inertial reference frame.
- An $i^{\text{th}}$ frame is sometimes denoted by $\mathbf{A}_{\text{i}}$.
- $\mathbf{A}_j^i$ sometimes denotes a frame $i$ described with respect to frame $j$.
- The following compact notation is used for trigonometric functions:

  $S_{ijk} = \sin(\theta_i + \theta_j + \theta_k)$ $\qquad$ $C_{ijk} = \cos(\theta_i + \theta_j + \theta_k)$
- **T** is generally used to denote transformations, while **H** is used for homogenous transformations.

### 2.1.4 Mathematical Preliminaries on Vectors and Matrices

A vector is defined with respect to a coordinate frame. Hence, a point can be described by different vectors defined in different coordinate frames, for instance, in Fig. 2.4. Vectors **A** and **B** show the same point but are basically different since **A** is described with respect to the $X_1Y_1Z_1$ coordinate frame and **B** is described with respect to the $X_2Y_2Z_2$ coordinate frame.

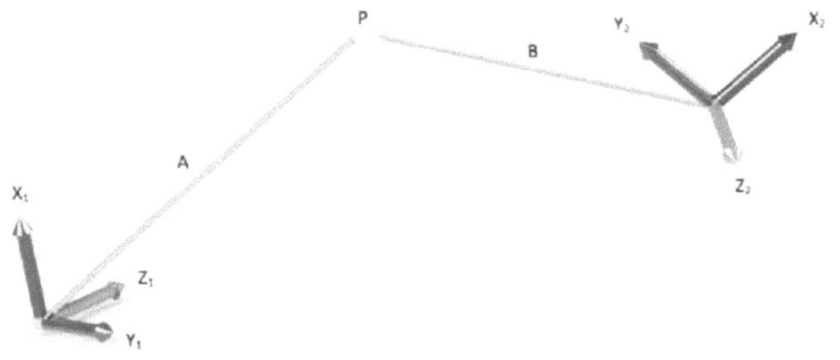


**Figure 2.4** Description of the same point in two different coordinate frames.

For vectors we use the standard notation, for example

$$\mathbf{a} \equiv \mathbf{a}_i \equiv [\mathrm{a}_1\mathrm{a}_2\mathrm{a}_3]^{\mathrm{T}} \tag{2.1}$$

In the Cartesian coordinate system *XYZ*, if the unit vectors along *X*, *Y* and *Z* are $\mathbf{e}_1$, $\mathbf{e}_2$, and $\mathbf{e}_3$, respectively, we can define the vector **a** as follows:

$$\mathbf{a} = \mathrm{a}_1\mathbf{e}_1 + \mathrm{a}_2\mathbf{e}_2 + \mathrm{a}_3\mathbf{e}_3 \tag{2.2}$$

The dot product of two vectors **a** and **b** is the multiplication of the magnitude of one of the vectors by the magnitude of the projection of the other one on the prior vector and is defined such that

$$\mathbf{a}\cdot\mathbf{b} = \mathrm{a}_1\mathrm{b}_1 + \mathrm{a}_2\mathrm{b}_2 + \mathrm{a}_3\mathrm{b}_3 \tag{2.3}$$

which equals $|\mathbf{a}|\cdot|\mathbf{b}|\cdot\cos\theta$, where $\theta$ is the angle between vectors **a** and **b**, and || stands for the absolute value of a vector.

The cross product of two vectors **a** and **b** is defined as the normal vector to the plane that includes both **a** and **b**, and its magnitude is $|\mathbf{a}|\cdot|\mathbf{b}|\cdot\sin\theta$, where $\theta$ is the angle between the two vectors. It is mathematically defined as or its vector form is

$$\mathbf{a}\times\mathbf{b} = \begin{vmatrix} \mathbf{e}_1 & \mathbf{e}_2 & \mathbf{e}_3 \\ \mathrm{a}_1 & \mathrm{a}_2 & \mathrm{a}_3 \\ \mathrm{b}_1 & \mathrm{b}_2 & \mathrm{b}_3 \end{vmatrix} = (\mathrm{a}_2\mathrm{b}_3 - \mathrm{a}_3\mathrm{b}_2)\mathbf{e}_1$$

$$-(\mathrm{a}_1\mathrm{b}_3 - \mathrm{a}_3\mathrm{b}_1)\mathbf{e}_2 + (\mathrm{a}_1\mathrm{b}_2 - \mathrm{a}_2\mathrm{b}_1)\mathbf{e}_3 \tag{2.4}$$

Multiplication of matrices is significantly used in both direct and inverse kinematics. The following shows how two matrices are multiplied:

$$\mathbf{b} = \mathbf{Aa} = \begin{bmatrix} A_{11} & A_{12} & A_{13} \\ A_{21} & A_{22} & A_{23} \\ A_{31} & A_{32} & A_{33} \end{bmatrix} \cdot \begin{bmatrix} a_1 \\ a_2 \\ a_3 \end{bmatrix} = \begin{bmatrix} b_1 \\ b_2 \\ b_3 \end{bmatrix}$$

$$b_1 = A_{11}a_1 + A_{12}a_2 + A_{13}a_3 \quad (2.5)$$

$$b_2 = A_{21}a_1 + A_{22}a_2 + A_{23}a_3$$

$$b_3 = A_{31}a_1 + A_{32}a_2 + A_{33}a_3$$

For instance, assume that **A** and **a** are

$$\mathbf{a} = [-102]^{\mathrm{T}};\ \mathbf{A} = \begin{bmatrix} 1 & 3 & 0 \\ 2 & 1 & -1 \\ 4 & 1 & 0 \end{bmatrix} \quad (2.6)$$

Then

$$\mathbf{b} = \mathbf{Aa} = \begin{bmatrix} 1 & 3 & 0 \\ 2 & 1 & -1 \\ 4 & 1 & 0 \end{bmatrix} \cdot \begin{bmatrix} -1 \\ 0 \\ 2 \end{bmatrix} = \begin{bmatrix} -1 \\ -4 \\ -4 \end{bmatrix} \quad (2.7)$$

The transpose of a matrix $\mathbf{A}_{ij}$ is equal to $\mathbf{A}_{ji}$ such that the rows and columns change their roles. Therefore

$$\mathbf{A}_{ij}^{T} = \mathbf{A}_{ji} = \begin{bmatrix} A_{11} & A_{21} & A_{31} \\ A_{12} & A_{22} & A_{32} \\ A_{13} & A_{23} & A_{33} \end{bmatrix} \quad (2.8)$$

**Example**: Find the transpose of **A**, where

$$\mathbf{A} = \begin{bmatrix} 1 & 2 & 3 \\ 4 & 5 & 6 \\ 7 & 8 & 9 \end{bmatrix}$$

**Solution**: The **A** transpose is

$$\mathbf{A}^{\mathrm{T}} = \begin{bmatrix} 1 & 4 & 7 \\ 2 & 5 & 8 \\ 3 & 6 & 9 \end{bmatrix}$$

The inverse of a matrix $\mathbf{A}_{ij}$ is defined as $\mathbf{A}_{ji}^{-1}$ such that

$$\mathbf{A}\mathbf{A}^{-1} = \mathbf{I} \tag{2.9}$$

where **I** is the unitary matrix—a matrix whose off-diagonal elements are identically zero and whose diagonal elements are unity. For instance, a $3 \times 3$ unitary matrix is

$$\mathbf{I} = \begin{bmatrix} 1 & 0 & 0 \\ 0 & 1 & 0 \\ 0 & 0 & 1 \end{bmatrix}$$

Generally, the inverse of a matrix can be calculated as

$$\mathbf{A}_{ij}^{-1} = \frac{\text{Transpose}\left(\text{cofactor } \mathbf{A}_{ij}\right)}{\det \mathbf{A}_{ij}} \tag{2.10}$$

Therefore, to calculate the inverse of matrix **A**, we need to calculate the transpose of the cofactor matrix of **A** and its determinant. You can refer to linear algebra textbooks to learn how the cofactors of matrices and their determinants are calculated.

Calculation of the cofactor of a matrix and consequently its inverse is a time-consuming process. To make it simple, you can use mathematical software packages such as MATLAB, Mathematica, and Maple to easily obtain the inverse of matrices.

**Example**: Find the inverse of $\mathbf{A} = \begin{bmatrix} 1 & 3 & 0 \\ 2 & 1 & -1 \\ 4 & 1 & 0 \end{bmatrix}$.

**Solution**: Cofactor $\mathbf{A}_{ij} = \begin{bmatrix} 1 & -4 & -2 \\ 0 & 0 & 11 \\ -3 & 1 & -5 \end{bmatrix}$

Transpose(cofactor $\mathbf{A}_{ij}$) $= \begin{bmatrix} 1 & 0 & -3 \\ -4 & 0 & 1 \\ -2 & 11 & -5 \end{bmatrix}$, and the determinant of **A** is −11; therefore

$$\mathbf{A}_{ij}^{-1} = -\frac{1}{11} \cdot \begin{bmatrix} 1 & 0 & -3 \\ -4 & 0 & 1 \\ -2 & 11 & -5 \end{bmatrix}$$

Multiplication of **A** and the calculated $\mathbf{A}^{-1}$ results in a $3 \times 3$ unitary matrix.

### 2.1.5 Homogenous Representation of Points and Objects

Before describing the homogenous representation of objects, the concept of a homogenous vector should be introduced. Homogenous vectors have the same direction but different magnitudes and components. Figure 2.5 shows a number of homogenous vectors.

A vector has three components in space, namely, $X = a \cdot w$, $Y = b \cdot w$, and $Z = c \cdot w$, and can be shown as $[X\ Y\ Z\ w]^{\mathrm{T}}$, in which $w$ is the scaling factor. A similar definition for homogenous planes can be stated since planes can be represented by their outward normal vector.

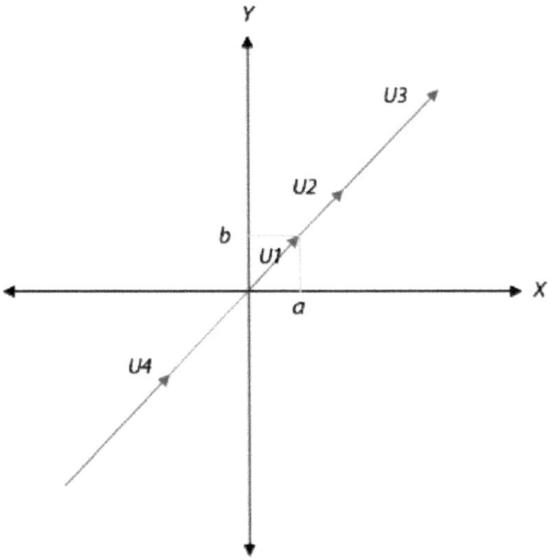


**Figure 2.5** Representation of homogenous vectors.

Points can be represented as homogenous position vectors such that a point **p** having coordinates $a$, $b$, and $c$ can be represented as a vector $\mathbf{u} = a\mathbf{i} + b\mathbf{j} + c\mathbf{k}$ and generally can be represented by

$\mathbf{u} = [X\ Y\ Z\ w]^T$, where $X = a{\cdot}w$, $Y = b{\cdot}w$, $Z = c{\cdot}w$, and $w$ is the scaling factor. Similarly, objects can be expressed as a set of points, that is, homogenous column vectors that normally are packed into a $4 \times n$ homogenous matrix, with $n$ representing the number of characteristic points peculiar to the object in a geometrical sense. For example, an inverted pyramid (Fig. 2.6) can be described easily by a $4 \times 5$ homogenous transformation.

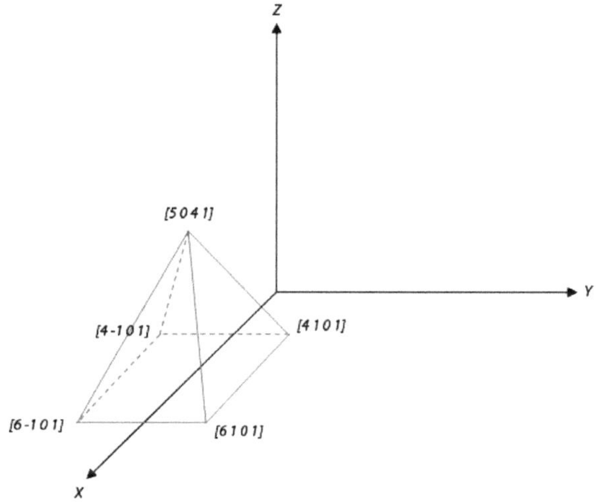


**Figure 2.6** Object representation by means of homogenous transformation made up of the object's homogenous characteristics.

Then the inverted pyramid can be represented by a homogenous transformation **A** such that

$$\mathbf{A} = \begin{bmatrix} 0 & 1 & -1 & -1 & 1 \\ 4 & 5 & 5 & 3 & 3 \\ 0 & 4 & 4 & 4 & 4 \\ 1 & 1 & 1 & 1 & 1 \end{bmatrix} \quad (2.11)$$

The order of appearance of columns in **A** is arbitrary. However, once set, it must remain the same. For example, the first column is the top vertex of the pyramid, and no matter what transformation the pyramid has undergone the first column will remain as the top vertex. Therefore, under a translation of $a$ units along the $a$ $x$ direction the proper transformation is

$$\mathbf{T}(x,a)=\begin{bmatrix}1&0&0&a\\0&1&0&0\\0&0&1&0\\0&0&0&1\end{bmatrix}$$

Oncethe transformation is applied to the inverted pyramid, it translates the pyramid along the direction by $a$ units and the new object is given by $\mathbf{A}_{\text{new}}$ such that

$$\mathbf{A}_{\text{new}}=\mathbf{T}\,\mathbf{A}=\begin{bmatrix}1&0&0&a\\0&1&0&0\\0&0&1&0\\0&0&0&1\end{bmatrix}\begin{bmatrix}0&1&-1&-1&1\\4&5&5&3&3\\0&4&4&4&4\\1&1&1&1&1\end{bmatrix}$$
$$=\begin{bmatrix}a&1+a&-1+a&-1+a&1+a\\4&5&5&3&3\\0&4&4&4&4\\1&1&1&1&1\end{bmatrix} \quad (2.12)$$

Now the pyramid top vertex or the first column is the point $[a401]$. Similar transformations may be applied to the object to rotate it around and translate it. However, all columns preserve their original identity as if we had labeled them with certain names such as *A*, *B*, C, *D*, and *E*.

### 2.1.6 Homogenous Transformations

A homogenous transformation is defined as a 4 × 4 matrix that generally represents translation, rotation, scaling, and perspective projection of points, vectors, and objects. It generally consists of a 3 × 3 rotation matrix, a 3 × 1 translation vector, a 1 × 3 perspective projection vector, and a 1 × 1 scaling matrix. Thus

$$\mathbf{T}=\begin{bmatrix}\text{Rotation}\,(3\times3)&\text{Translation}\,(3\times1)\\\text{Perspective projection}\,(1\times3)&\text{Scaling}\,(1\times1)\end{bmatrix} \quad (2.13)$$

Some important homogenous transformation matrices are given in Table 2.1.

**Table 2.1** Common homogenous transformations

**Rotation around the *X* coordinate by an angle $\alpha$:**

$$\text{Rotation}\ (X,\alpha)=\begin{bmatrix} 1 & 0 & 0 & 0 \\ 0 & \cos\alpha & -\sin\alpha & 0 \\ 0 & \sin\alpha & \cos\alpha & 0 \\ 0 & 0 & 0 & 1 \end{bmatrix} \tag{2.14}$$

**Rotation around the *Y* coordinate by an angle $\theta$:**

$$\text{Rotation}\ (Y,\theta)=\begin{bmatrix} \cos\theta & 0 & \sin\theta & 0 \\ 0 & 1 & 0 & 0 \\ -\sin\theta & 0 & \cos\theta & 0 \\ 0 & 0 & 0 & 1 \end{bmatrix} \tag{2.15}$$

**Rotation around the *Z* coordinate by an angle $\beta$:**

$$\text{Rotation}\ (Z,\beta)=\begin{bmatrix} \cos\beta & -\sin\beta & 0 & 0 \\ \sin\beta & \cos\beta & 0 & 0 \\ 0 & 0 & 1 & 0 \\ 0 & 0 & 0 & 1 \end{bmatrix} \tag{2.16}$$

**Transformation for *a* along the *X* axis, *b* along the *Y* axis, and *c* along the *Z* axis:**

$$\text{Translation}\ (a,b,c)=\begin{bmatrix} 1 & 0 & 0 & \boldsymbol{a} \\ 0 & 1 & 0 & \boldsymbol{b} \\ 0 & 0 & 1 & \boldsymbol{c} \\ 0 & 0 & 0 & 1 \end{bmatrix} \tag{2.17}$$

**Rotation around an arbitrary direction *K* by an angle $\theta$ ($K = k_1 i + k_2 j + k_3 k$):**

$$\text{Rotation}\ (K,\theta)=\begin{bmatrix} k_1\cdot k_1\cdot(1-\cos\theta)+\cos\theta & k_2\cdot k_1\cdot(1-\cos\theta)-k_3\cdot\sin\theta & k_3\cdot k_1\cdot(1-\cos\theta)+k_2\cdot\sin\theta & 0 \\ k_1\cdot k_2\cdot(1-\cos\theta)+k_3\cdot\sin\theta & k_2\cdot k_2\cdot(1-\cos\theta)+\cos\theta & k_3\cdot k_2\cdot(1-\cos\theta)-k_1\cdot\sin\theta & 0 \\ k_1\cdot k_3\cdot(1-\cos\theta)-k_2\cdot\sin\theta & k_2\cdot k_3\cdot(1-\cos\theta)+k_1\cdot\sin\theta & k_3\cdot k_3\cdot(1-\cos n)+\cos\theta & 0 \\ 0 & 0 & 0 & 1 \end{bmatrix} \tag{2.18}$$

**Example**: Find the homogenous transformation that moves the pyramid in Fig. 2.6 to the position illustrated in Fig. 2.7.

**Solution**: As you can see in the figures, the object undergoes a translation for 1 unit along the $X$ axis, a rotation around the $X$ axis by 180°, a rotation around the $Z$ axis by –90°, and a translation along the $Z$ axis for –4 units, respectively. Negative signs are movements in negative directions.
Thus,
**H** = Translation ($X$, 1). Rotation ($X$, 180°). Rotation ($Z$, –90°). Translation ($Z$, –4)

Each of the terms in the above equation can be easily obtained as mentioned previously; therefore

$$\mathbf{H}=\begin{bmatrix}1&0&0&1\\0&1&0&0\\0&0&1&0\\0&0&0&1\end{bmatrix}\cdot\begin{bmatrix}1&0&0&0\\0&-1&0&0\\0&0&-1&0\\0&0&0&1\end{bmatrix}\cdot\begin{bmatrix}0&1&0&0\\-1&0&0&0\\0&0&1&0\\0&0&0&1\end{bmatrix}\cdot\begin{bmatrix}1&0&0&0\\0&1&0&0\\0&0&1&-4\\0&0&0&1\end{bmatrix}$$

Then

$$\mathbf{H}=\begin{bmatrix}0&1&0&1\\1&0&0&0\\0&0&-1&4\\0&0&0&1\end{bmatrix} \tag{2.19}$$

And the new positions of vectors are

$$\mathbf{A}_{\text{new}}=\mathbf{HA}=\begin{bmatrix}0&1&0&1\\1&0&0&0\\0&0&-1&4\\0&0&0&1\end{bmatrix}\cdot\begin{bmatrix}0&1&-1&-1&1\\4&5&5&3&3\\0&4&4&4&4\\1&1&1&1&1\end{bmatrix} \tag{2.20}$$

$$\mathbf{A}_{\text{new}}=\begin{bmatrix}5&6&6&4&4\\0&1&-1&-1&1\\4&0&0&0&0\\1&1&1&1&1\end{bmatrix}$$

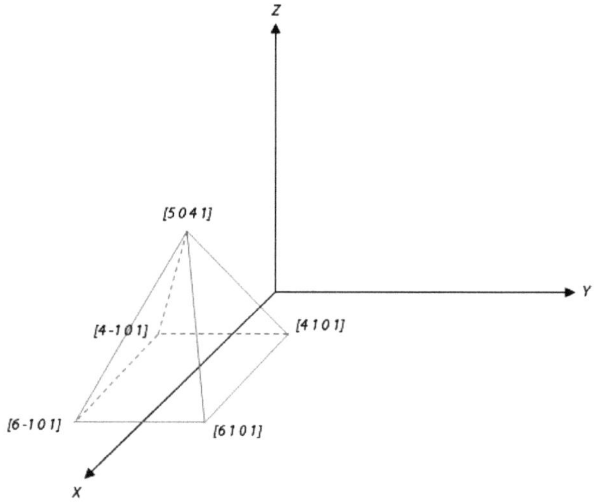


**Figure 2.7** Object manipulation

## 2.1.7 Robotic Manipulator Joint Coordinate Systems

A manipulator consists of a series of links connected by a series of joints. Homogenous transformations with respect to local joint coordinates are called **A** matrices (i.e., D–H transformations). Let $\mathbf{A}_1$ describe the position and orientation of the first link with respect to the base, $\mathbf{A}_2$ that of the second link with respect to the first link, $\mathbf{A}_3$ that of the third link with respect to the second link, and so on. Then the position and orientation of the $n^{\text{th}}$ link with respect to the base coordinate will be

$$\mathbf{T}_n = \mathbf{A}_1\mathbf{A}_2\mathbf{A}_3 \ldots \mathbf{A}_{n-1}\mathbf{A}_n \tag{2.21}$$

The products of **A** matrices are called **T** matrices.$\mathbf{T}_n$ is designated the end-effector transformation, such that the end-effector origin has a position vector **p**. Attached to the origin is a rectangular Cartesian coordinate system whose orientation designates the orientation of the end effector. For any link joint coordinate $i$, the link direction at the joint is in the approach vector direction ($\mathbf{a}_i$), the direction of the link-to-link rotation is in the $\mathbf{o}_i$ direction (the orientation vector), and the normal unit vector $\mathbf{n}_i$ forms a right-handed system with $\mathbf{o}_i$ and $\mathbf{a}_i$. The position vector of this $i^{\text{th}}$ joint with respect to the base coordinate is $\mathbf{p}_i$, thus, the transformation $\mathbf{T}_i$ of this joint coordinate is

$$\mathbf{T}_i = \begin{bmatrix} n_{ix} & o_{ix} & a_{ix} & p_{ix} \\ n_{iy} & o_{iy} & a_{iy} & p_{iy} \\ n_{iz} & o_{iz} & a_{iz} & p_{iz} \\ 0 & 0 & 0 & 1 \end{bmatrix} \quad (2.22)$$

### 2.1.8 Denavit–Hartenberg Representations

As defined previously, a generalized robotic arm may be considered a kinematic chain interconnected at joints whose motions can be servo-controlled by proper actuators. The interconnections are either revolute (rotary) or prismatic (telescopic) or a combination of the two. Figure 2.8 depicts a number of common robotic joints.

In 1955, Denavit and Hartenberg defined the concept of a "lower pair" joint as the one created by contacting surfaces. In this sense, "upper pair" joints are the ones created by either point or line contacts between two bodies. Thus, in Fig. 2.8, the joints (a), (b), (c), (d), (e), and (f) are lower pairs, while the joints (g), (h), (i), and (j) are upper pairs.

Now consider a pair of adjacent robotic links interconnected by lower pairs capable of rotation and telescopic motion (Fig. 2.9). The coordinates are chosen as follows:

1. The $\boldsymbol{Z}_i$ axis is along the axis of motion or rotation of the $i + 1^{\text{th}}$ joint.
2. The $\boldsymbol{X}_i$ axis is in the direction normal to both the $\boldsymbol{Z}_i$ and $\boldsymbol{Z}_{i-1}$ axes, pointing away from the $\boldsymbol{Z}_{i-1}$ axis (such as to make a right-handed coordinate with either $\boldsymbol{Z}_i$ and $\boldsymbol{Z}_{i-1}$ or $\boldsymbol{Z}_{i-1}$ and $\boldsymbol{Z}_i$).
3. The $\boldsymbol{Y}_i$ coordinate is chosen so as to make the $X_i Y_i Z_i$ coordinate system a right-handed coordinate system.
4. The distance between the two common normals $a_i$ and $a_{i-1}$ is called the link distance $d_i$.
5. The length of the normal $a_i$ is the minimum distance between the $\boldsymbol{Z}_i$ and $\boldsymbol{Z}_{i-1}$ axes. If this is zero, the direction of $a_i$ becomes arbitrary. Note that $a_i$ is also referred to as the length of the $i^{\text{th}}$ link.
6. The relative orientation of the $\boldsymbol{X}_i$ axis with respect to the $\boldsymbol{X}_{i-1}$ axis is called $\theta_i$ or the vector of the joint angles.

7. The relative orientation of the $\boldsymbol{Z}_i$ axis with respect to the $\boldsymbol{Z}_{i-1}$ axis is called $\alpha_i$ or the vector of twist angles.

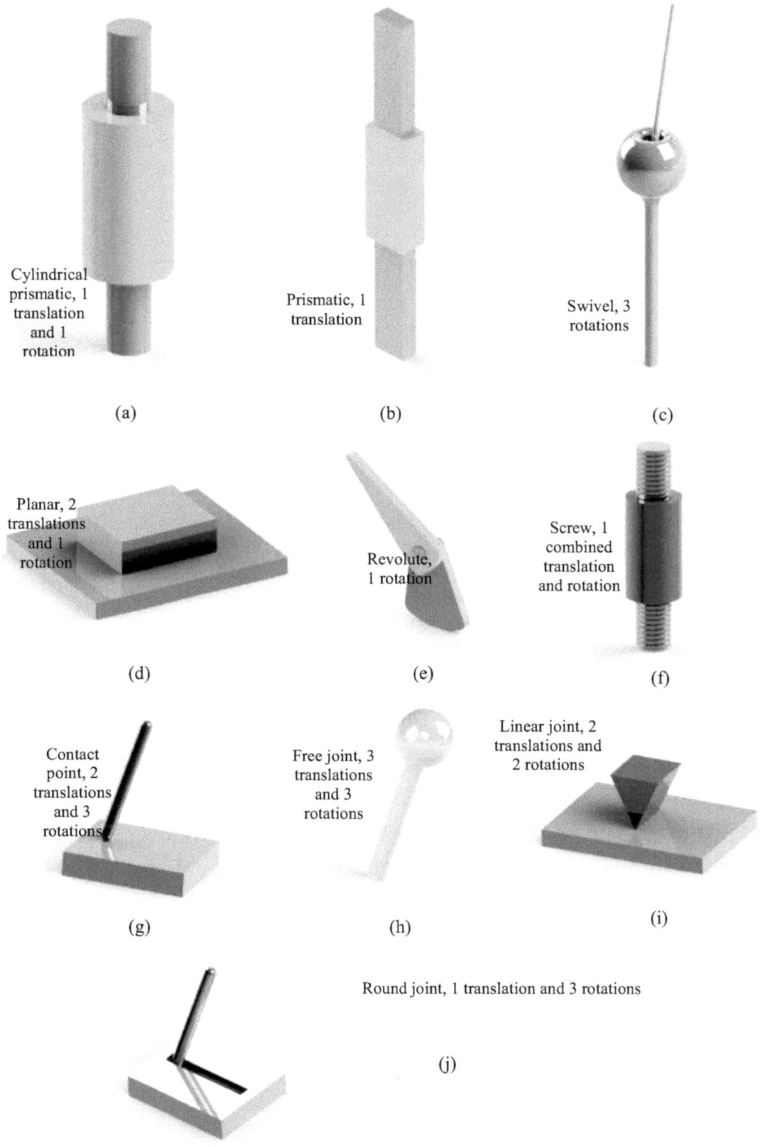


**Figure 2.8** General schematic description of robotic joints.

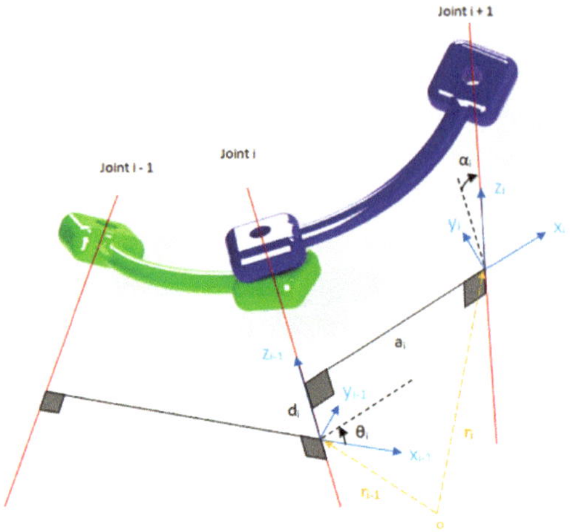


**Figure 2.9** Generalized robotic link coordinate systems.

The four parameters $d_i$, $\theta_i$, $a_i$, and $\alpha_i$ constitute a minimally sufficient set to determine the kinematic configuration of each link of the robotic arm. Note that $d_i$ is the joint distance, $\theta_i$ is the joint angle, $a_i$ is the link length, and $\alpha_i$ is the link twist angle. For a plane revolute joint, generally $d_i$, $a_i$, and $\alpha_i$ are all constant, while $\theta_i$ varies as link $i$ rotates about the axis of joint $i$. On the other hand, for a prismatic joint, $\theta_i$, $a_i$, and $\alpha_i$ are constant, while $d_i$ varies as link $i$ slides along the axis of joint $i$. Thus, for both cases, $a_i$ and $\alpha_i$ are generally constant and depend on the design of the robot. For example, when the joint axes of adjacent joints intersect, then the link length $a$ is also zero (such is the case with prismatic joints).

Once the D–H coordinate system for each link is established, a homogenous transformation matrix can be developed easily, relating the $i^{\text{th}}$ coordinate frame. Referring to Fig. 2.7, we can see that a point expressed in the $i^{\text{th}}$ coordinate system may be expressed in the $i - 1^{\text{th}}$ coordinate system by performing the following successive transformations:

1. A rotation around the $\boldsymbol{Z}_{i-1}$ axis by an angle $\theta_i$ to align the $\boldsymbol{X}_{i-1}$ and $\boldsymbol{X}_i$ axes
2. A translation along the $\boldsymbol{Z}_{i-1}$ axis for a distance $d_i$ to bring the $\boldsymbol{X}_{i-1}$ and $\boldsymbol{X}_i$ axes
3. A translation along $\boldsymbol{X}_i$ axis for a distance $a_i$ to bring the two origins into coincidence

4. A rotation around the $\boldsymbol{X}_i$ axis by an angle $\alpha_i$ to make the two coordinate systems completely coincide

Thus, the complete transformation of link $i$ with respect to link $i$ $-1$ or joint $i$ with respect to joint $i-1$ is
$\mathbf{H}_{i-1}^{i} = \mathbf{T}_{i-1}^{i} = \mathbf{A}_{i-1}^{i}$ = Rotation$(Z_{i-1}, \theta_i)$. Translation $(Z_{i-1}, d_i)$. Translation $(X_i, a_i)$. Rotation $(X_i, \alpha_i)$
or

$$\mathbf{A}_{i-1}^{i} = \begin{bmatrix} \cos\alpha_i & -\sin\alpha_i & 0 & 0 \\ \sin\alpha_i & \cos\alpha_i & 0 & 0 \\ 0 & 0 & 1 & 0 \\ 0 & 0 & 0 & 1 \end{bmatrix} \cdot \begin{bmatrix} 1 & 0 & 0 & 0 \\ 0 & 1 & 0 & 0 \\ 0 & 0 & 1 & d_i \\ 0 & 0 & 0 & 1 \end{bmatrix} \cdot \begin{bmatrix} 1 & 0 & 0 & a_i \\ 0 & 1 & 0 & 0 \\ 0 & 0 & 1 & 0 \\ 0 & 0 & 0 & 1 \end{bmatrix}$$

$$\begin{bmatrix} 1 & 0 & 0 & 0 \\ 0 & \cos\alpha_i & -\sin\alpha_i & 0 \\ 0 & \sin\alpha_i & \cos\alpha_i & 0 \\ 0 & 0 & 0 & 1 \end{bmatrix}$$

$$\mathbf{A}_{i-1}^{i} = \mathbf{A}_i = \begin{bmatrix} \cos\theta_i & -\cos\alpha_i.\sin\theta_i & \sin\alpha_i.\sin\theta_i & a_i.\cos\theta_i \\ \sin\theta_i & \cos\alpha_i.\cos\theta_i & -\sin\alpha_i.\cos\theta_i & a_i.\sin\theta_i \\ 0 & \sin\alpha_i & \cos\alpha_i & d_i \\ 0 & 0 & 0 & 1 \end{bmatrix} \tag{2.23}$$

$\mathbf{A}_i$ shows the transformation pertaining to the $i^{\text{th}}$ link. Furthermore, if $\boldsymbol{r}_i$ is the homogenous coordinate of the $i^{\text{th}}$ joint and $\boldsymbol{r}_{i-1}$ is the homogenous coordinate of the $i$–$1^{\text{th}}$ joint, it is clear that

$$\boldsymbol{r}_{i-1} = \mathbf{A}_{i-1}^{i}.\boldsymbol{r}_i \tag{2.24}$$

The following algorithm completely assigns and establishes link coordinate systems compatible with D–H transformations for a given $n$-degree-of-freedom robotic arm. Adjacent links can be related to each other kinematically through a set of $4 \times 4$ homogenous transformation matrices. The first coordinate system pertaining to the base is denoted by a homogenous system $[X_0Y_0Z_01]^{\text{T}}$ at the supporting base. The origin of this system is denoted as the $0^{\text{th}}$ joint.

1. Establish the base coordinate $X_0Y_0Z_0$ such that the $\boldsymbol{Z_0}$ axis lies along the axis of motion of joint 1.
2. Initialize and loop for each $i = 1, 2, ..., n$.
3. Align all $\boldsymbol{Z_i}$ with the axis of motion or rotation of joint $i + 1$.
4. Establish the origin of the $i^{\text{th}}$ coordinate system either at the intersection of the $\boldsymbol{Z_i}$ and $\boldsymbol{Z_{i-1}}$ axes or at the intersection of the common normal between the $\boldsymbol{Z_i}$ and $\boldsymbol{Z_{i-1}}$ axes.
5. Establish $\boldsymbol{X_i}$ at each $i^{\text{th}}$ joint, either by $\pm(\boldsymbol{Z_{i-1}} \times \boldsymbol{Z_i})$ or along the common normal between $\boldsymbol{Z_{i-1}}$ and $\boldsymbol{Z_i}$ when they are parallel.
6. Establish the $\boldsymbol{Y_i}$ axis by $\boldsymbol{Y_i} = +(\boldsymbol{Z_i} \times \boldsymbol{X_i})$ to complete the right-handed coordinate system.
7. Find $d_i$ as the distance from the origin of the $i{-}1^{\text{th}}$ coordinate system to the intersection of the $\boldsymbol{Z_{i-1}}$ axis and the $\boldsymbol{X_i}$ axis.
8. Find $\alpha_i$ as the distance from the intersection of the $\boldsymbol{Z_{i-1}}$ and $\boldsymbol{X_i}$ axes to the origin of the $i^{\text{th}}$ coordinate system.
9. Find $\theta_i$ as the angle of rotation from the $\boldsymbol{X_{i-1}}$ axis to the $\boldsymbol{X_i}$ axis.
10. Find $\alpha_i$ as the angle of rotation from the $\boldsymbol{Z_{i-1}}$ axis to the $\boldsymbol{Z_i}$ axis about the $\boldsymbol{Z_i}$ axis.

In prismatic joints, the $\boldsymbol{Z}$ axis can also be established parallel to the actuation direction for ease of calculations.

**Example:** Do the direct and inverse kinematics of the robotic arm depicted in Fig. 2.10.

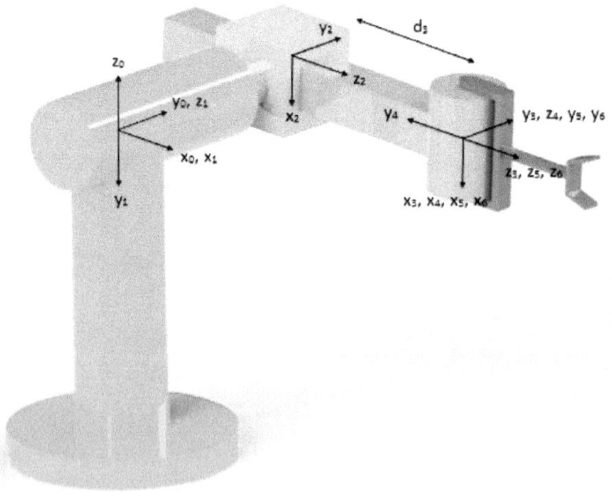


**Figure 2.10** A cylindrical robotic manipulator.

**Solution**: This robotic arm consists of one telescopic motion and five rotary motions. Moreover, there are two rolling motions involved before and after the pitch motion to assist the robotic arm in simulating the yaw motion. The joint coordinate systems are shown in the figure. Note that in the following, $S_i = \sin\theta_i$ and $C_i = \cos\theta_i$:

$$\mathbf{A}_0^1 = \begin{bmatrix} C_1 & 0 & -S_1 & 0 \\ S_1 & 0 & C_1 & 0 \\ 0 & -1 & 0 & 0 \\ 0 & 0 & 0 & 1 \end{bmatrix}; \quad \mathbf{A}_0^1 = \begin{bmatrix} C_1 & 0 & -S_1 & 0 \\ S_1 & 0 & C_1 & 0 \\ 0 & -1 & 0 & 0 \\ 0 & 0 & 0 & 1 \end{bmatrix};$$

$$\mathbf{A}_2^3 = \begin{bmatrix} 1 & 0 & 0 & 0 \\ 0 & 1 & 0 & 0 \\ 0 & 0 & 1 & d_3 \\ 0 & 0 & 0 & 1 \end{bmatrix}; \quad \mathbf{A}_3^4 = \begin{bmatrix} C_4 & 0 & -S_4 & 0 \\ S_4 & 0 & C_4 & 0 \\ 0 & -1 & 0 & 0 \\ 0 & 0 & 0 & 1 \end{bmatrix};$$

$$\mathbf{A}_4^5 = \begin{bmatrix} C_5 & 0 & S_5 & 0 \\ S_5 & 0 & -C_5 & 0 \\ 0 & 1 & 0 & 0 \\ 0 & 0 & 0 & 1 \end{bmatrix}; \quad \mathbf{A}_5^6 = \begin{bmatrix} C_6 & -S_6 & 0 & 0 \\ S_6 & C_6 & 0 & 0 \\ 0 & 0 & 1 & 0 \\ 0 & 0 & 0 & 1 \end{bmatrix}$$

To find $\mathbf{T}_0^6$, multiply the above matrices, we have

$$\mathbf{T}_0^6 = \mathbf{A}_0^1 \cdot \mathbf{A}_1^2 \cdot \mathbf{A}_2^3 \cdot \mathbf{A}_3^4 \cdot \mathbf{A}_4^5 \cdot \mathbf{A}_5^6 = \begin{bmatrix} n_x & o_x & a_x & p_x \\ n_y & o_y & a_y & p_y \\ n_z & o_z & a_z & p_z \\ 0 & 0 & 0 & 1 \end{bmatrix} \quad (2.25)$$

$\mathbf{T}_0^6$ matrix elements can easily be calculated, we have

$$n_x = C_1[C_2(C_4C_5C_6 - S_4S_6) - S_2S_5S_6] - S_1(S_4C_5C_6 + C_4C_6), \quad (2.26)$$

$$n_y = S_1[C_2(C_4C_5C_6 - S_4S_6) - S_2S_5S_6] + C_1(S_4C_5C_6 + C_4C_6), \quad (2.27)$$

$$n_z = -S_2\,(C_4C_5C_6 - S_4S_6) - C_2S_5S_6, \quad (2.28)$$

$$o_x = C_1[-C_2(C_4C_5C_6 - S_4S_6) - S_2S_5S_6] - S_1(-S_4C_5C_6 + C_4C_6), \tag{2.29}$$

$$o_y = S_1[-C_2(C_4C_5C_6 - S_4S_6) - S_2S_5S_6] + C_1(-S_4C_5S_6 + C_4C_6), \tag{2.30}$$

$$o_z = S_2(C_4C_5C_6 + S_4S_6) + S_2S_5S_6, \tag{2.31}$$

$$a_x = C_1(C_2C_4C_5 + S_2S_5) - S_1S_4S_5, \tag{2.32}$$

$$a_y = S_1(C_2C_4C_5 + S_2C_5) + C_1S_4S_5, \tag{2.33}$$

$$a_z = -S_2C_4C_5 + C_4C_5, \tag{2.34}$$

$$p_x = C_1S_2d_3 - S_1d_2, \tag{2.35}$$

$$p_y = S_1S_2d_3 + C_1d_2, \text{ and} \tag{2.36}$$

$$p_z = C_2d_3, \tag{2.37}$$

There are 12 equations that relate joint parameters to the position and orientation of the end effector and vice versa. If the joint parameters are known, the position and orientation of the end effector can be easily obtained using the above 12 equations. However, if we know the position and orientation of the end effector and want to calculate the joint parameters, we have to solve the above-mentioned equations for $\theta_1$, $\theta_2$, ..., $\theta_6$. This process is called inverse kinematics analysis. To solve these equations, some mathematical prerequisites are essential, which are beyond the scope of this book. In the following topics, inverse kinematic analysis is illustrated through simpler problems.

### 2.1.9 Direct and Inverse Kinematics in Robotics

In the *n*-degrees-of-freedom robotic arm, **A**s can be calculated and multiplied in order to obtain the $\mathbf{T}_n$ matrix. $\mathbf{T}_n$ shows the relative position and orientation of the end-effector coordinate frame with respect to the base coordinate, which is a function of joint parameters, $\boldsymbol{\theta_1} = [\theta_1\ \theta_2\ \theta_3 ... \theta_n]^{\mathrm{T}}$.

If joint parameters are known in a robotic arm, $\mathbf{T}_n$ can be calculated with the help of D–H transformation. In other words, the relative position and orientation of the robotic arm end effector with respect to the base coordinate frame can be shown as a function of the joint parameters. This procedure is called the direct kinematic analysis of robotic manipulators.

If the relative position and orientation of the robotic arm end effector with respect to the base are known, the joint parameters to lead to that position and orientation can be calculated by solving a set of trigonometric equations obtained from D–H transformation analysis. This process is called the inverse kinematic analysis of robotic manipulators.

The inverse kinematic analysis of robotic arms is more applicable to engineering problems. For instance, to perform intraocular robotic surgery, a special point in the eye has to be reached at a specific orientation; therefore, knowing what combination of joint parameters leads the robotic arm to that position and orientation seems necessary.

Aside from the D–H method to analyze the kinematic attitude of robotic arms, geometrical relationships between the robotic links can be employed to perform direct and inverse kinematic analysis. This is shown in the following examples.

**Example:** Do the direct and inverse kinematics of the robotic arm depicted in Fig. 2.11.

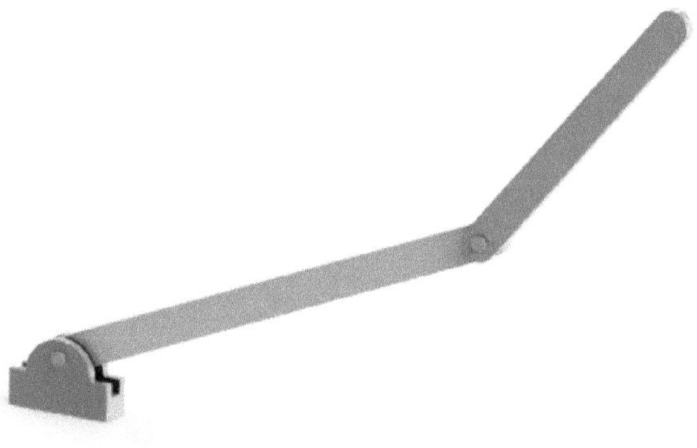

**Figure 2.11** A two-link robotic manipulator.

**Solution**: The following trigonometric equations can be easily obtained from Fig. 2.12. All the constants are illustrated in Fig. 2.12. We have

$$X = l_1C_1 + l_2C_{12}$$

$$Y = l_1S_1 + l_2S_{12}$$

This is the direct kinematic analysis of a two-link robotic arm. Now we solve these two equations for $\theta_2$. First we take the square of both sides of each of the equations above:

$$X^2 = l_1^2 \cdot C_1^2 + l_2^2 \cdot C_{12}^2 + 2l_1 \cdot l_2 \cdot C_1 \cdot C_{12}$$

$$Y^2 = l_1^2 \cdot S_1^2 + l_2^2 \cdot S_{12}^2 + 2l_1 \cdot l_2 \cdot S_1 \cdot S_{12}$$

Add these equations:

$$X^2 + Y^2 = l_1^2 \cdot (S_1^2 + C_1^2) + l_1^2 \cdot (S_{12}^2 + C_{12}^2) + 2l_1 \cdot l_2 \cdot (C_1 \cdot C_{12} + S_1 \cdot S_{12})$$

Thus

$$X^2 + Y^2 - l_1^2 + l_2^2 + 2l_1 \cdot l_2 \cdot C_2$$

$$C_2 = \frac{X^2 + Y^2 - l_1{}^2 - l_2{}^2}{2.\,l_1.\,l_2} = a*$$

$$S_2 = \sqrt{1 - a*^2}$$

$$\tan\theta_2 = \frac{\sqrt{1 - a^{*2}}}{a^*}$$

$$\theta_2 = \tan^{-1}\left(\frac{\sqrt{1 - a^{*2}}}{a^*}\right)$$

or

$$\theta_2 = \tan^{-1}\left(\frac{\sqrt{4.\,l_1^2.\,l_2^2 - \left(X^2 + Y^2 - l_1{}^2 - l_2{}^2\right)^2}}{X^2 + Y^2 - l_1{}^2 - l_2{}^2}\right) \tag{2.38}$$

We also know from the geometry of the two-link robot (Fig. 2.12) that

$$\theta_1 = \phi - \theta = \tan^{-1}\left(\frac{Y}{X}\right) - \tan^{-1}\left(\frac{p}{q}\right)$$

Thus

$$\theta_1 = \tan^{-1}\left(\frac{Y}{X}\right) - \tan^{-1}\left(\frac{l_2\,.\,S_2}{l_1 + l_2\,.\,C_2}\right) \tag{2.39}$$

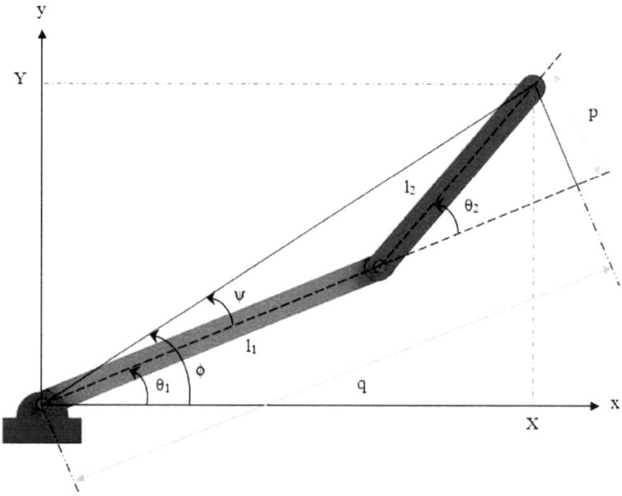


**Figure 2.12** A two-link robotic manipulator's geometrical properties.

Using the inverse kinematic solution of the two-link robotic manipulator, we can calculate the joint parameters ($\theta_1$, $\theta_2$) if we know the geometrical constants and position of the end effector ($l_1$, $l_2$, $X$, $Y$). Therefore, we know how much to actuate the joint actuators in order to reach a specific position.

**Example:** Determine the joint parameters in both two-link robotic arms shown in Fig. 2.13 so that they keep the rectangular object in a specific position ($a$, $b$) at an angle $\theta$.

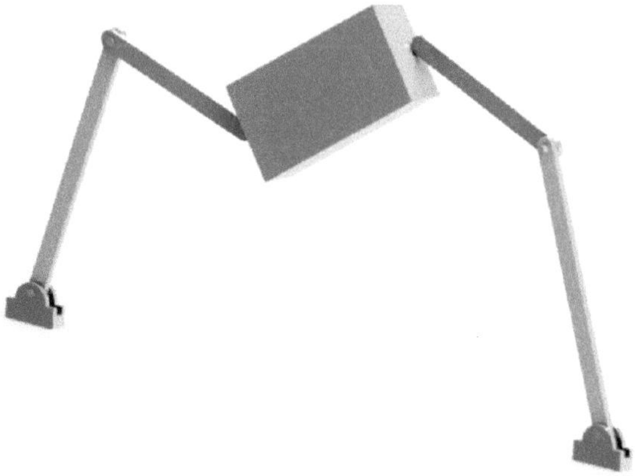

**Figure 2.13** Two two-link robotic arms manipulating an object.

We assume that the object is a homogenous rectangle $w \times s$, and the center of mass is in the middle (Fig. 2.14). The origin of the $X_1Y_1$ coordinate system is at $(X_1, 0)$, and the origin of the $X_2Y_2$ coordinate system is at $(X_1 + d, 0)$.

From Fig. 2.14, it is clear that the tip positions $p$ and $q$ are given by

$$p = \left(a + \frac{w}{2} \cdot \cos\theta\right)\boldsymbol{i} + \left(b + \frac{w}{2} \cdot \sin\theta\right)\boldsymbol{j}$$

$$q = \left(a - \frac{w}{2} \cdot \cos\theta\right)\boldsymbol{i} + \left(b - \frac{w}{2} \cdot \sin\theta\right)\boldsymbol{j}$$

In the $XY$ coordinate system, $P$ is at $\left(a + \frac{w}{2} \cdot \cos\theta, b + \frac{w}{2} \cdot \sin\theta\right)$, and therefore, the location of $p$ in the $X_2Y_2$ coordinate system is $\left(a + \frac{w}{2} \cdot \cos\theta - \mathrm{X}_1 - d, b + \frac{w}{2} \cdot \sin\theta\right)$.

In the $XY$ coordinate system, $q$ is at $\left(a - \frac{w}{2} \cdot \cos\theta, b - \frac{w}{2} \cdot \sin\theta\right)$, and therefore, the location of $q$ in the $X_1Y_1$ coordinate system is $\left(a - \frac{w}{2} \cdot \cos\theta - \mathrm{X}_1, b - \frac{w}{2} \cdot \sin\theta\right)$.

Now we solve two inverse kinematics problems separately. For the left two-link robotic arm, we know the position of $q$ with respect to the $X_1Y_1$ coordinate system. Thus, we can easily determine $\psi$. This also holds for the right arm.

We already solved the inverse kinematics problem of a two-link robotic arm. We just need to use the solution of the previous example and substitute new constants into it. We have the following:

*The left two-link robotic arm*:

$l_1 = l_{11}$

$l_1 = l_{12}$

$X = a - \frac{w}{2} \cdot \cos\theta - X_1$ ⟹ We now substitute these into the equations obtained in the previous example

$$X = a - \frac{w}{2} \cdot \cos\theta - X_1$$

$$\theta_1 = \theta_{11}$$

$$\theta_2 = \theta_{12}$$

$$\theta_{12} = \tan^{-1}\left( \frac{\sqrt{4 \cdot l_{11}^2 \cdot l_{12}^2 - \left( \left( a - \frac{w}{2} \cdot \cos\theta - X_1 \right)^2 + (b - \frac{w}{2} \cdot \sin\theta)^2 - {l_{11}}^2 - {l_{12}}^2 \right)^2}}{\left( a - \frac{w}{2} \cdot \cos\theta - X_1 \right)^2 + (b - \frac{w}{2} \cdot \sin\theta)^2 - {l_{11}}^2 - {l_{12}}^2} \right) \tag{2.40}$$

$$\theta_{11} = \tan^{-1}\left( \frac{b - \frac{w}{2} \cdot \sin\theta}{a - \frac{w}{2} \cdot \cos\theta - X_1} \right) - \tan^{-1}\left( \frac{l_{12} \cdot \sin\theta_{12}}{l_{11} + l_{12} \cdot \cos\theta_{12}} \right) \tag{2.41}$$

*The right two-link robotic arm*:

$$l_1 = l_{21}$$

$$l_2 = l_{22}$$

$$\mathrm{X} = a + \frac{w}{2} \cdot \cos\theta - \mathrm{X}_1 - d \Longrightarrow$$

We now substitute these into the equations obtained in the previous example

$$Y = b + \frac{w}{2} \cdot \sin\theta$$

$$\theta_1 = \theta_{21}$$

$$\theta_2 = \theta_{22}$$

$$\theta_{22} = \tan^{-1}\left(\frac{\sqrt{4 . l_{21}^2 . l_{22}^2 - \left(\left(a+\frac{w}{2}.\cos\theta - X_1 - d\right)^2 + (b+\frac{w}{2}.\sin\theta)^2 - {l_{21}}^2 - {l_{22}}^2\right)^2}}{\left(a+\frac{w}{2}.\cos\theta - X_1 - d\right)^2 + (b+\frac{w}{2}.\sin\theta)^2 - {l_{21}}^2 - {l_{22}}^2}\right) \tag{2.42}$$

$$\theta_{21} = \tan^{-1}\left(\frac{b+\frac{w}{2}.\sin\theta}{a+\frac{w}{2}.\cos\theta - X_1 - d}\right) - \tan^{-1}\left(\frac{l_{22} . \sin\theta_{22}}{l_{21} + l_{22} . \cos\theta_{12}}\right) \tag{2.43}$$

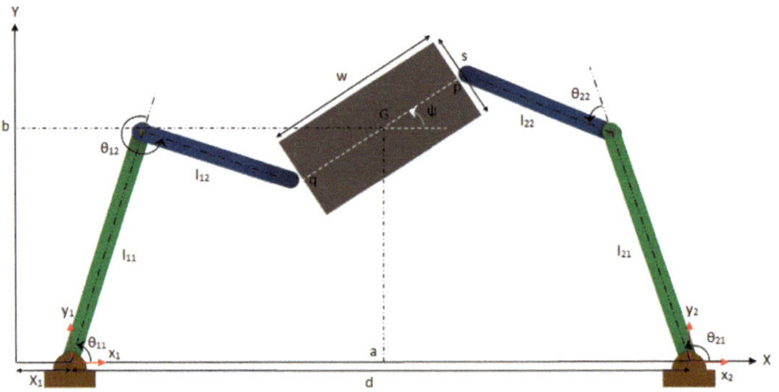


**Figure 2.14** Geometrical properties of two two-link robotic arms.

If we want to keep a rectangular object in a specific position with a specific orientation by using two two-link robotic arms, we can easily calculate the joint parameters ($\theta_{11}$, $\theta_{12}$, $\theta_{21}$, $\theta_{22}$) from the above equations and consequently actuate the actuators properly to reach that position.

## 2.2 Robotic Workspace

The workspace of a robotic manipulator is defined as the set of all 3D points that can be reached by a reference point located on the robotic hand. A restricted version of a robotic workspace is also defined as the set of all points that can be reached by a fixed orientation of the robotic hand. The knowledge of robotic workspaces is important in arranging the associated surgical tools, personnel, objects, and devices around the surgical robot and assessing the efficiency of the operating room in which the surgical robot is located. In general, the boundary of a robotic workspace, which is called the robotic work envelope, is a complex surface difficult to represent explicitly by geometrical equations. To derive mathematical expressions for robotic work surfaces, we customarily employ the D–H homogeneous transformations to describe the locus of the trajectories produced by the robotic hand. Seeking analytical solutions for the workspace of a robotic manipulator is a tedious task. However, by means of numerical methods, we can easily get an understanding of the workspace of a robotic arm. For example, consider the 2D two-link robotic arm shown in Fig. 2.15. The position of the tip of the robot can be expressed by the following equations:

$$X = l_1 . \cos\theta_1 + l_2 . \cos(\theta_1 + \theta_2)$$

$$Y = l_1 . \sin\theta_1 + l_2 . \sin(\theta_1 + \theta_2)$$

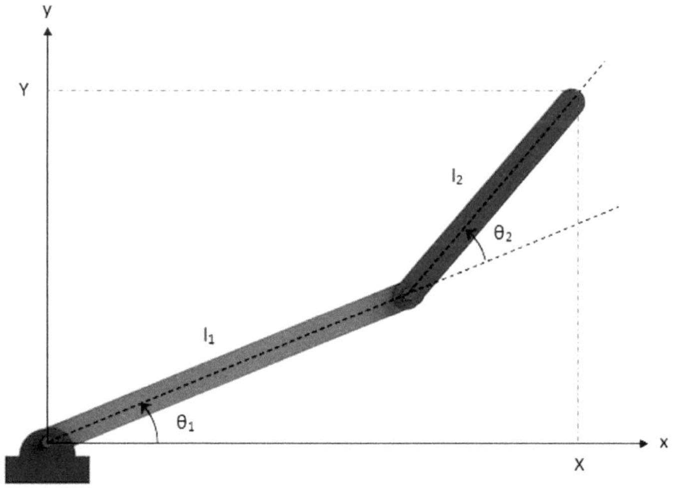


**Figure 2.15** A 2D two-link robotic manipulator.

The lengths of these two links are constant, while $\theta_1$ and $\theta_2$ are the only variables. We can easily employ numerical analysis software such as MATLAB to draw the cloud of the tip positions with all the possible set of incremental variables.

For the two-link robotic arm depicted in Fig. 2.15 with the following constants and constraints, the workspace is as illustrated in Fig. 2.16 (for MATLAB codes refer to appendix A):

$l_1 = 40; l_2 = 15$

$$0 \le \theta_1 \le 90; 0 \le \theta_2 \le 90$$

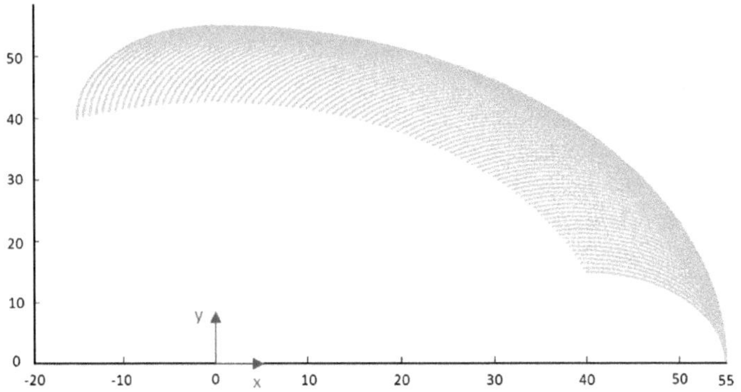


**Figure 2.16** The two-link robotic manipulator workspace; case 1.

Also, with the following constants and constraints, the workspace is as shown in Fig. 2.17:

$l_1 = 40; l_2 = 15$

$$0 \le \theta_1 \le 270; 0 \le \theta_2 \le 90$$

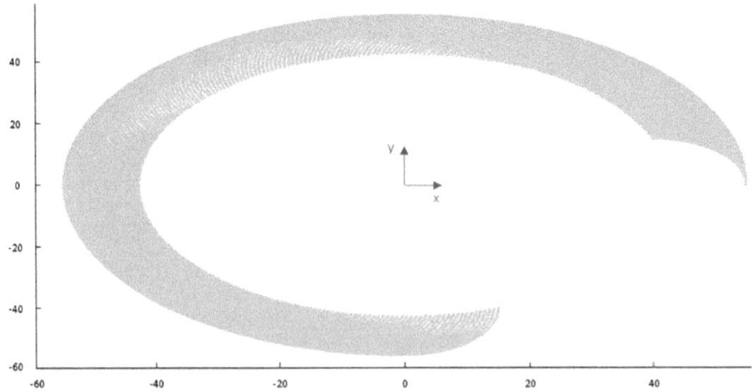


**Figure 2.17** The two-link robotic manipulator workspace; case 2.

In a 2D three-link robotic manipulator with the following constants and constraints, the workspace is as illustrated in Fig. 2.18:

$l_1 = 40; l_2 = 15; l_3 = 5$

$0 \leq \theta_1 \leq 180; 0 \leq \theta_2 \leq 90; 0 \leq \theta_3 \leq 90$

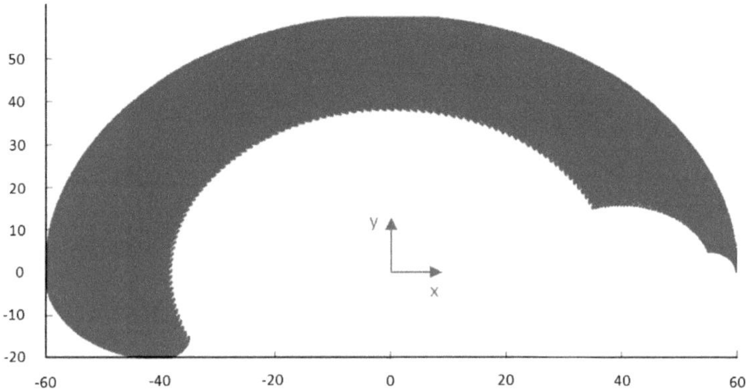


**Figure 2.18** The three-link robotic manipulator workspace; case 1.

Also, with the following constants and constraints, the workspace is as shown in Fig. 2.19:

$l_1 = 40; l_2 = 15; l_3 = 5$

$0 \leq \theta_1 \leq 90; 0 \leq \theta_2 \leq 90; 0 \leq \theta_3 \leq 90$

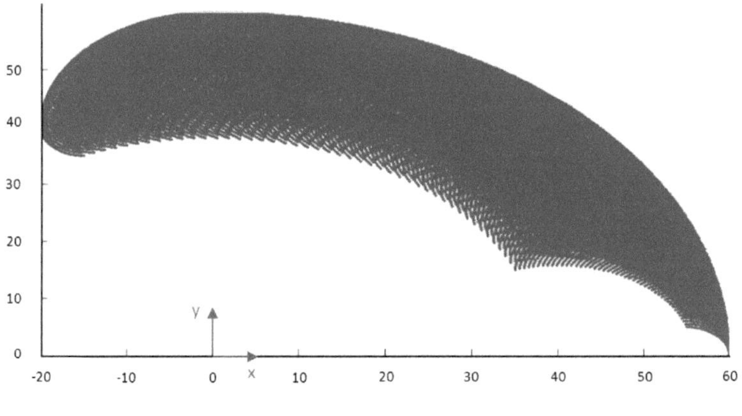


**Figure 2.19** The three-link robotic manipulator workspace; case 2.

In a 2D four-link robotic manipulator with the following constants and constraints, the workspace is as illustrated in Fig. 2.20:

$l_1 = 40; l_2 = 15; l_3 = 5; l_4 = 5$

$0 \leq \theta_1 \leq 40; 0 \leq \theta_2 \leq 90; 0 \leq \theta_3 \leq 90; 0 \leq \theta_4 \leq 20$

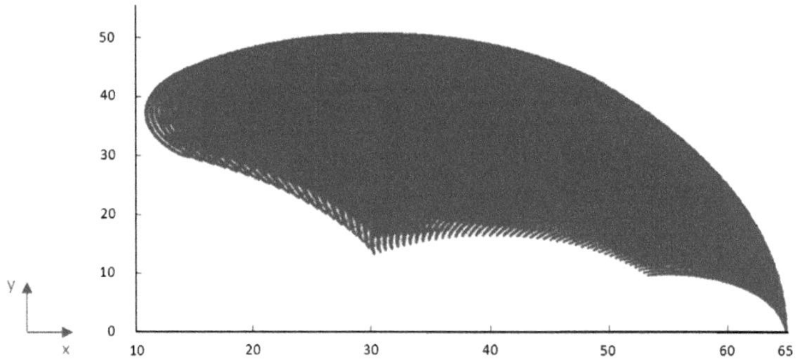


**Figure 2.20** The four-link robotic manipulator workspace.

If the two-link robotic manipulator base is placed on a vertical pole so that it can travel up and down, then we have a 3D problem. The workspace in this case can be calculated numerically using the same method, which is shown in Fig. 2.21:

$l_1 = 40; l_2 = 15$

$0 \leq \theta_1 \leq 90; 0 \leq \theta_2 \leq 90 \qquad 0 \leq z \leq 100$

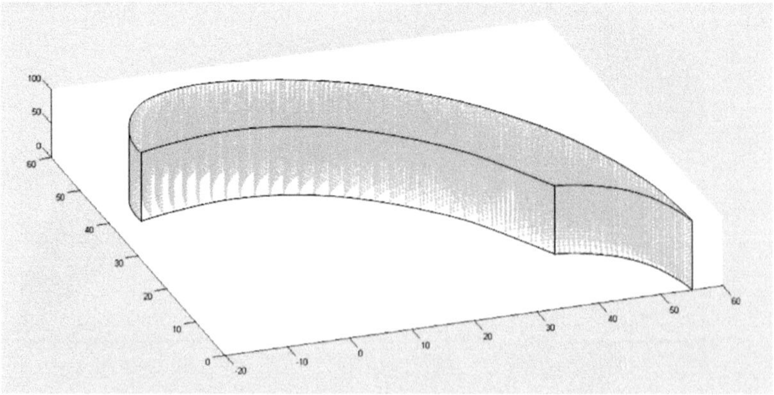

**Figure 2.21** The 3D two-link robotic manipulator workspace.

## 2.3 Robotic Trajectory

We must concern ourselves with the techniques of motion trajectory design for surgical robots. We need to describe the desired motion of robotic manipulators in the joint space, the 3D workspace, or the hand coordinates, in as much as the time histories of position, orientation, linear velocity, angular velocity, linear acceleration, and angular acceleration are concerned. For instance, in a pick-and-place robotic system, the mission is to pick an object from one location and place it in another. However, we might need to program the robotic system in more detail. There may be some obstacles in the way of the robotic hand, which we must avoid to prevent collision. Thus, what path the robotic manipulator hand takes to perform its eventual mission is important. To design the trajectory of a robotic hand we need to define the functionality of joint parameters with each other.

For example, in a three-link planar robotic manipulator if we constrain the joint parameters with different functions we get different trajectories of the tip of the arm, as shown in Fig. 2.22 (for MATLAB codes refer to appendix A).

$l_1 = 40; l_2 = 15; l_3 = 5$

$\theta_1 = \theta_1$

$\theta_2 = \theta_1 \cdot \sin(5\theta_1)$

$\theta_3 = \theta_1 \cdot \cos(7\theta_1)$

$0 \le \theta_1 \le 90$

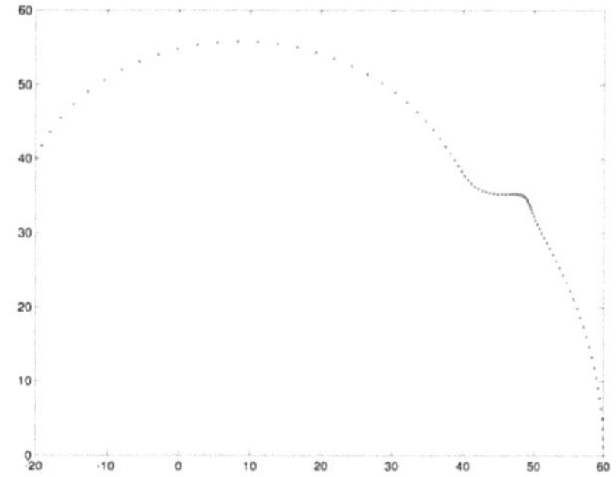

(a)

$l_1 = 40; l_2 = 15; l_3 = 5$

$\theta_1 = \theta_1$

$\theta_2 = \theta_1 \cdot \sin(3\theta_1)$

$\theta_3 = \theta_1 \cdot \cos(2\theta_1)$

$0 \le \theta_1 \le 90$

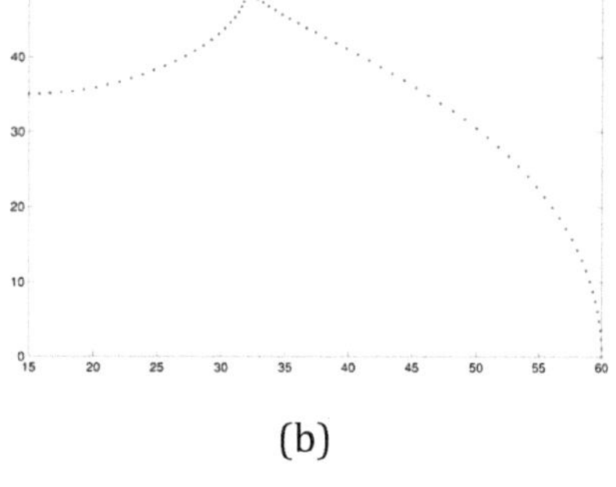

(b)

$l_1 = 40; l_2 = 15; l_3 = 5$
$\theta_1 = \theta_1$
$\theta_2 = \theta_1 \cdot \sin(3\theta_1)$
$\theta_3 = \theta_1 \cdot \cos(4\theta_1)$
$0 \leq \theta_1 \leq 90$

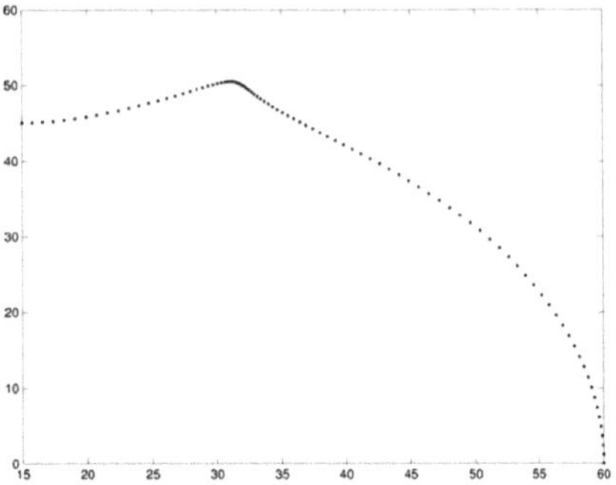

(c)

$l_1 = 40; l_2 = 15; l_3 = 5$
$\theta_1 = \theta_1$
$\theta_2 = \theta_1 \cdot \sin(-2\theta_1)$
$\theta_3 = \theta_1 \cdot \cos(6\theta_1)$
$0 \leq \theta_1 \leq 90$

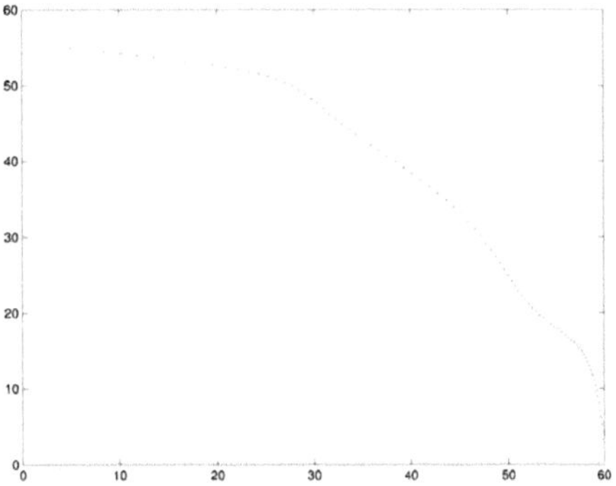

(d)

$l_1 = 40; l_2 = 15; l_3 = 5$
$\theta_1 = \theta_1$
$\theta_2 = \theta_1 \cdot \tan(-2\theta_1)$
$\theta_3 = \theta_1 \cdot \cos(6\theta_1)$
$0 \leq \theta_1 \leq 40$

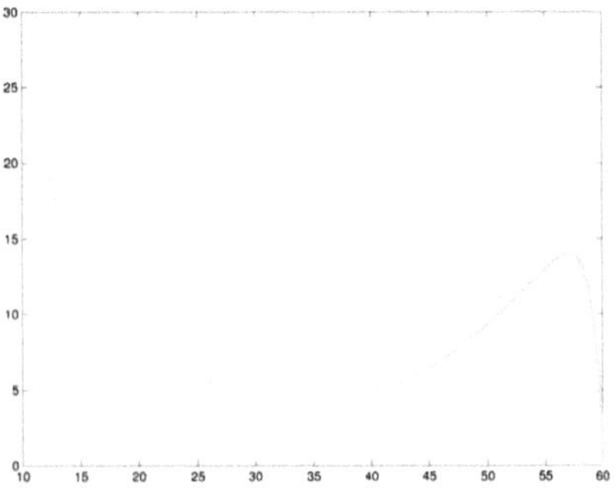

(e)

$$l_1 = 40; l_2 = 15; l_3 = 5$$

$$\theta_1 = \theta_1$$

$$\theta_2 = -\theta_1^{\frac{1}{\theta_1}}$$

$$\theta_3 = \theta_1 \cdot \cos(6\theta_1)$$

$$0 \le \theta_1 \le 40$$

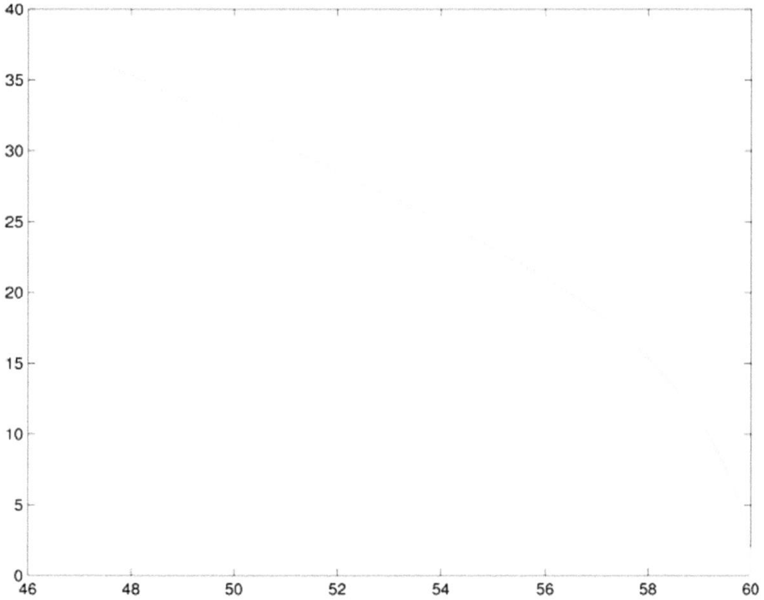


**Figure 2.22** Different tip trajectories of a three-link robotic arm under different joint parameter constraints.

In Fig. 2.23 $\theta_2$ s and $\theta_3$s were different functions of $\theta_1$s and we illustrated how different functionalities resulted in different trajectories. This process can be done the other way around. We can define the functionality of joint parameters such that a point set on a robotic arm follows a special trajectory. This requires higher-level mathematics knowledge and is more than the level this book is intended for.

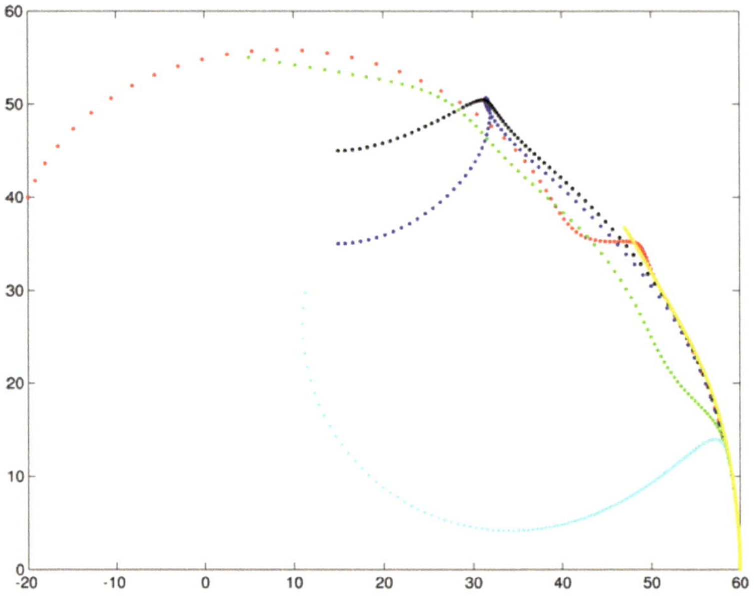


**Figure 2.23** Combined tip trajectories of the three-link robotic arm shown in Fig. 2.22, all illustrated in one picture for comparison.

## Problem Set

1. What are "kinematics" and "kinematics of robotic manipulators"?
2. Describe "robotic manipulators".
3. Mathematically, how is the position and orientation of a robotic end-effector described?
4. Describe "direct kinematics" and "inverse kinematics".
5. What are "homogenous transformations"?
6. Describe "lower pair joint" and "upper pair joint".
7. What are the steps in establishing link coordinate systems compatible with D-H transformations for a given *n*-degree of freedom robotic arm?
8. Define "robotic workspace".
9. Perform the direct kinematic analysis of the surgical system shown in the following picture.

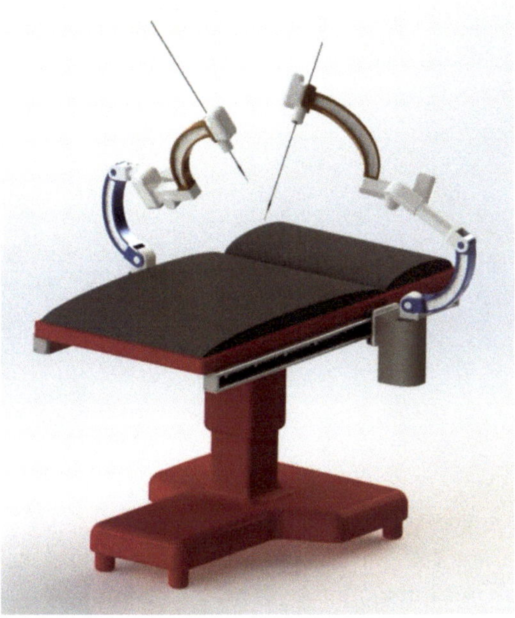

10. Generate X-Y workspace of the robotic surgical system shown in problem 9 at a number of arbitrary Zs.

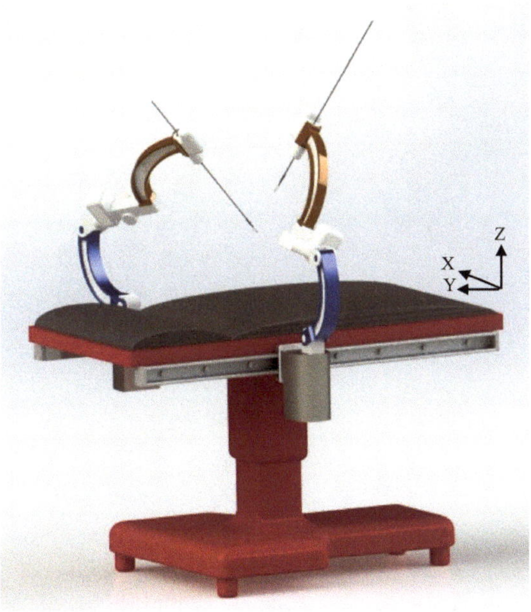

11. Perform the direct kinematic analysis of the WAM robotic hand shown in the following picture.

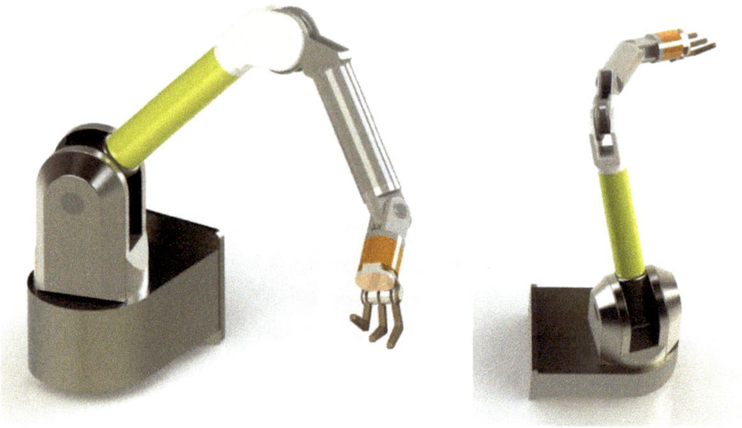

12. Generate Y-Z workspace of the WAM robotic hand shown in problem 11 at a number of arbitrary Xs.

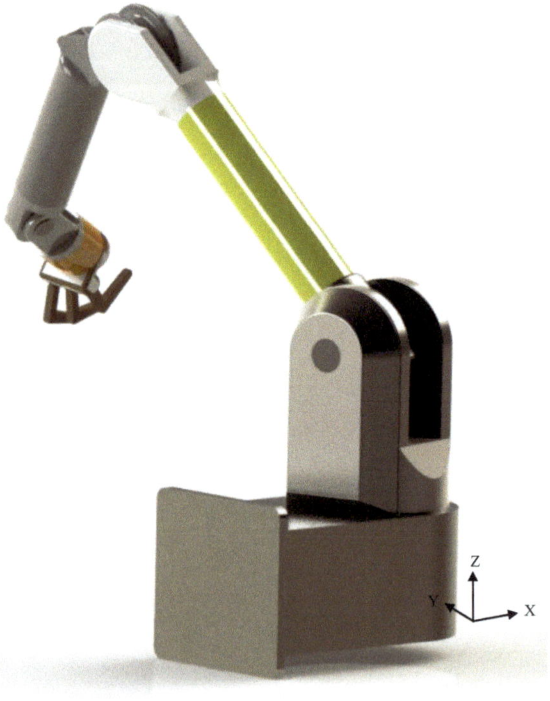

13. Perform the direct kinematic analysis of the surgical system shown in the following picture.

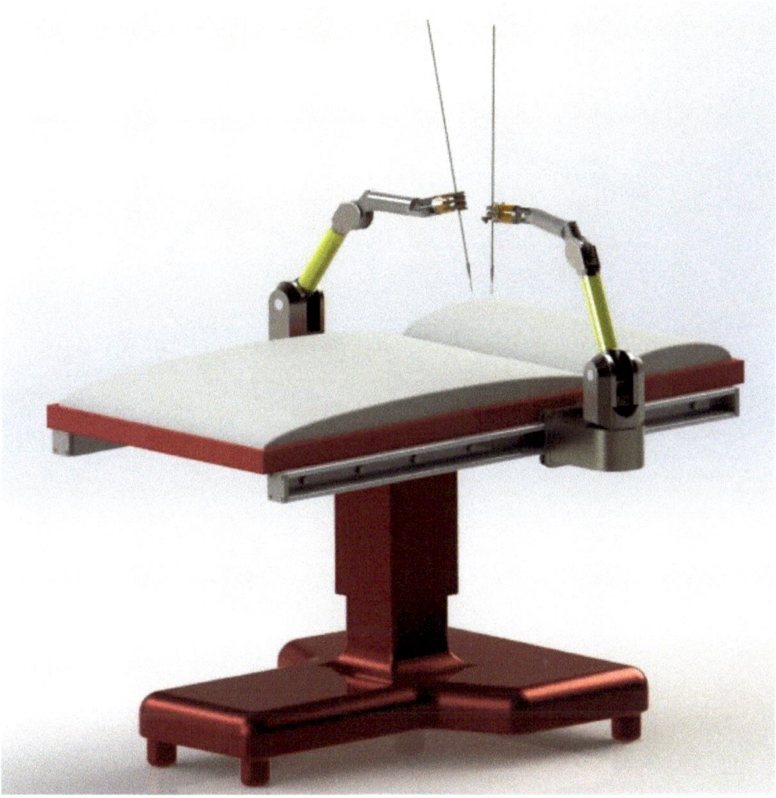

14. Generate X-Z workspace of the robotic surgical system shown in problem 13 at a number of arbitrary Ys.

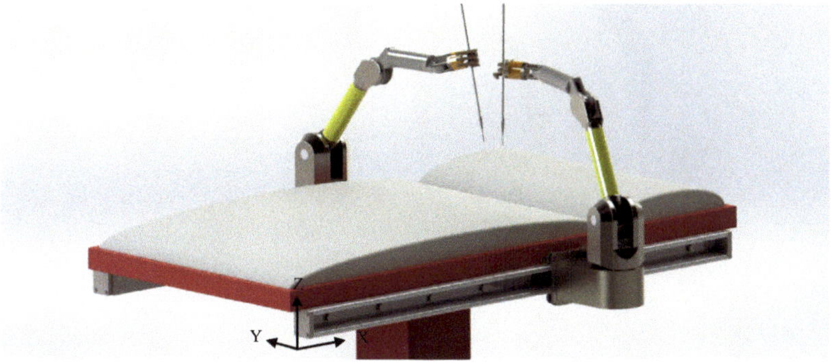

15. Perform the direct kinematic analysis of the surgical system shown in the following picture.

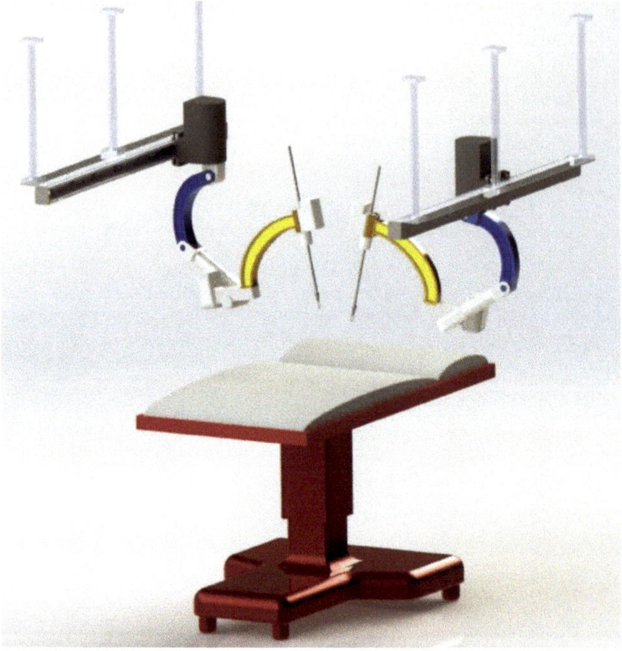

16. Generate Y-Z workspace of the robotic surgical system shown in problem 15 at a number of arbitrary Xs.

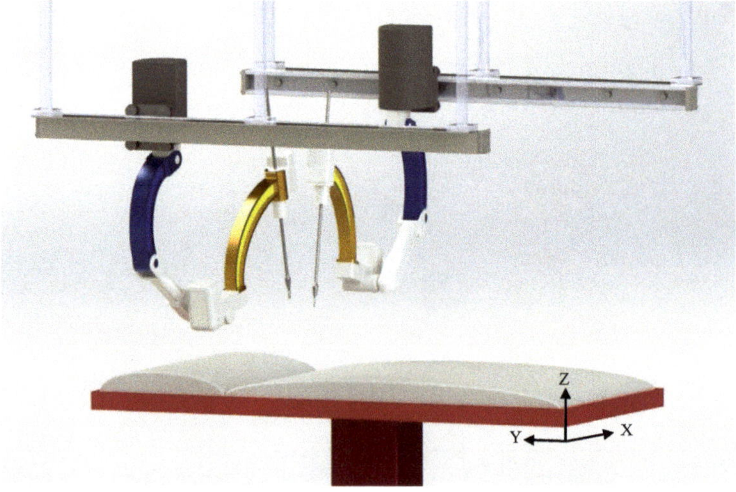

17. Perform the direct kinematic analysis of the surgical system shown in the following picture.

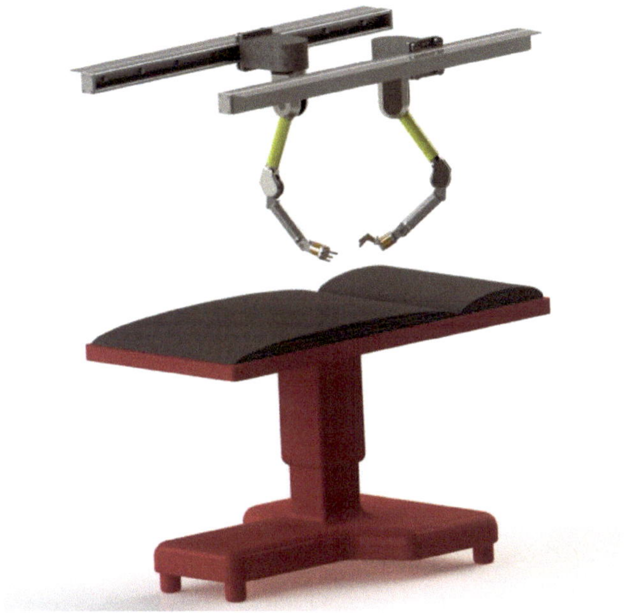

18. Generate X-Z workspace of the robotic surgical system shown in problem 17 at a number of arbitrary Ys.

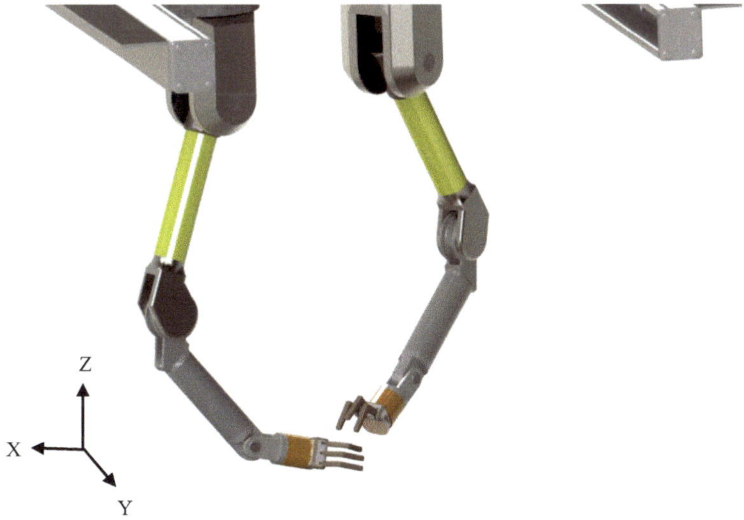

# Chapter 3

# Intraocular Robotic Surgical System

## 3.1 Introduction to Ophthalmic Surgery

Ophthalmic surgery is any type of operation that is performed on the eye, the anatomy of which is shown in Fig. 3.1. Eyes are sensitive organs, and their surgical workspace is relatively small. Thus, higher precision is required when performing ocular surgical operations as compared to surgeries on other organs. There are limitations on the surgeons' hand precision. Their hands may also fail in making precise moves during long surgeries. Introduction of robots for ophthalmic surgeries can solve this issue. Intraocular surgery involves various types of eye surgery, such as glaucoma surgery, refractive surgery, corneal surgery, vitreoretinal surgery, eye muscle surgery, oculoplastic surgery, eyelid removal, orbital removal, eye removal, and cataract removal, some which are briefly described next.

- *Cataract surgery.* Cataracts are a result of metabolic changes in crystalline lens fibers of the eyes—more specifically, denaturation of the lens protein—and cause loss of visual acuity and contrast sensitivity. Although aging is a typical cause for development of cataracts and they are common among elderly people, they may also occur by exposure to ultraviolet light, entry of toxic materials into the eye, diseases

*Robotic Surgery: Smart Materials, Robotic Structures, and Artificial Muscles*
Mohsen Shahinpoor and Siavash Gheshmi

ISBN 978-981-4316-23-1 (Hardcover), 978-981-4463-51-5 (eBook)
www.panstanford.com

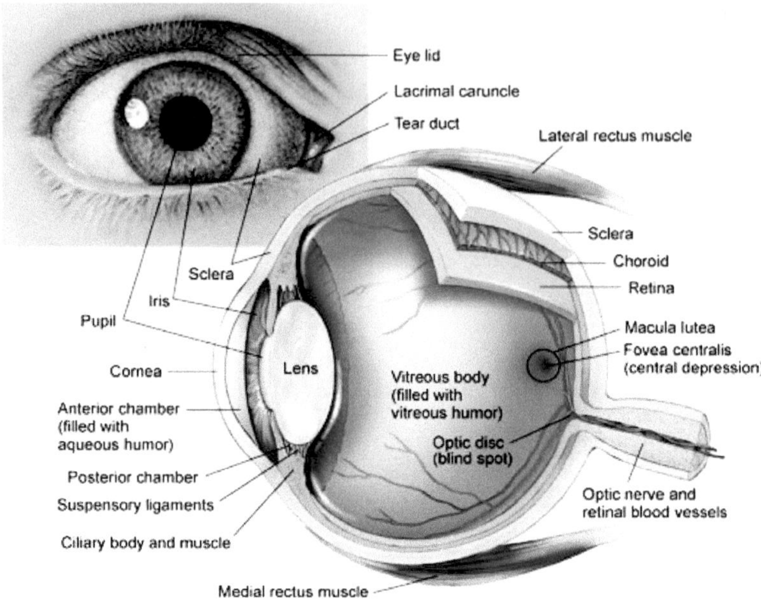


**Figure 3.1** Right eye anatomy (viewed from above).[1]

like diabetes, etc. This problem can also be congenital. There are both nonsurgical and surgical methods to treat cataracts. Nonsurgical methods suggest application of eyedrops if the cataract is not fully developed. However, fully developed cataracts imply surgical treatments during which the natural lens of the eye is removed and replaced with an artificial intraocular lens (IOL).

- *Glaucoma surgery.* Successive loss of vision and eventual blindness can occur when the optic nerve is damaged by a type of eye disease referred to as glaucoma. The aqueous fluid produced inside the eye globe flows around and eventually leaves the eye through the anterior chamber. When extra aqueous fluid is produced or less aqueous fluid than necessary is drained, the intraocular pressure (IOP) increases, impeding the blood flow to the optical nerve and causing damage to it. High IOP is recognized as the main cause for glaucoma. Laser and conventional surgeries are offered as temporary solutions to treat glaucoma, as there is no cure for it yet.

[1]http://www.biographixmedia.com/human/eye-anatomy.html

- *Refractive surgery.* This term refers to any surgery performed on the eye to improve its refractive state. Cataract surgery can also be referred to as a refractive surgery because it enhances refraction in the eye by implanting an artificial IOL. However, it is mostly related to cases when the cornea is reshaped to provide better visual acuity. Lasers are a great tool for performing this type of operation, commonly known as laser-assisted intraocular keratotomy (LASIK).
- *Vitreoretinal surgery.* This term refers to any ophthalmic surgery performed to treat problems related to the retina, macula, and vitreous fluid, such as retinal detachment and diabetic retinopathy.
- *Eye muscle surgery.* Eye muscles control the movement of the eye globe, as shown in Fig. 3.2. They move the eyes in all directions to cover a large vision area. Eye muscle surgery can become necessary to treat diseases related to the alignment of eyes, such as strabismus. Eye muscles are strengthened, weakened, or repositioned during the course of such an operation.

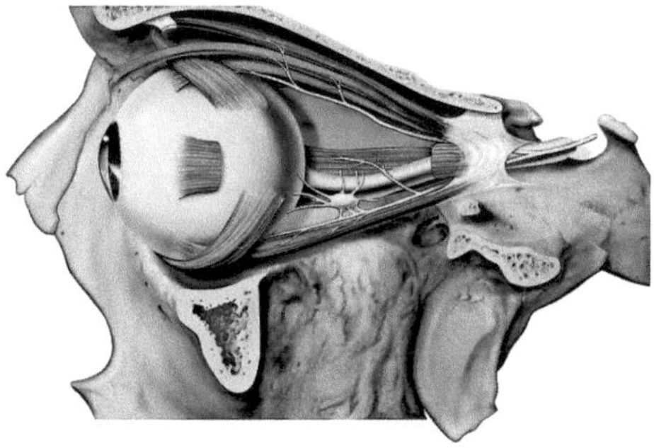

**Figure 3.2** Muscles of the left orbit.[2]

- *Oculoplastic surgery.* This is also known as corrective, cosmetic, and reconstructive surgery. While the focus of most ophthalmic surgeries is the eyeball itself, this surgical operation is concerned with the tissue and anatomic structures surrounding the eye, such as the orbit, eyelids, and tear ducts.

---

[2]http://en.wikipedia.org/wiki/Muscles_of_orbit

Ophthalmic surgery is not limited to the aforementioned categories and includes more types such as corneal surgery and eye removal. In the following section, a history of robotics in ocular surgeries is provided.

## 3.2 Robot-Assisted Intraocular Surgery

Robotic surgery has proved to be useful in surgeries operated in confined spaces. Intraocular surgery, which demands precision manipulation of surgical instruments, an excellent technical skill set, the least tremor, and a high degree of visualization, is no exception. Several robotic systems have been introduced and developed for use in microsurgeries. Meenink et al. (2010) discuss the benefits of a master-slave robot for vitreoretinal eye surgery, which is shown in Fig. 3.3. This robotic system is used to perform surgeries on the inner side at the back of the eye, for example, the vitreous humor and the retina. They claim that the advantages of this system are a comfortable body posture, intuitive instrument handling, downscaled instrument movements, upscaled force feedback, and filtering of hand tremor.

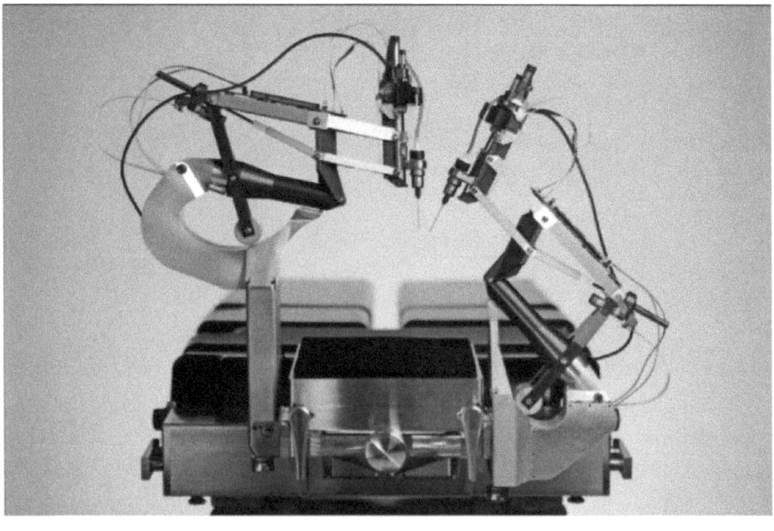

**Figure 3.3** Robotic system developed by Meenink et al. (2010).

Sutherland et al. (2006) introduced a robotic system for use in microsurgical operation. This system, which is shown in Fig. 3.4, includes two six-degrees-of-freedom movable arms, which are carried on a wheeled base. These arms are equipped with special end effectors and actuators to be able to manipulate different surgical tools. A magnetic resonance imaging (MRI) experiment is used to digitize the position of the tool tip relative to fiducial markers. They further developed their system, and in 2012 they introduced an enhanced version of their system. In the new version, robotic arms include a magnetic resonance (MR)-compatible structural material, multiple MR-compatible joint motors, and multiple MR-compatible joint encoders.

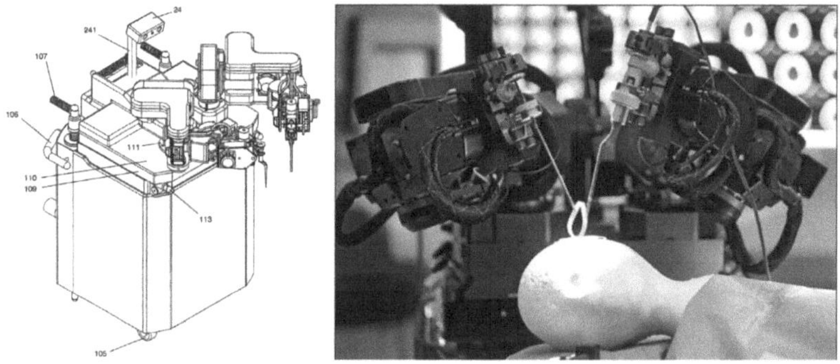

(a) (b)

**Figure 3.4** Robotic system developed by Sutherland et al. (2006). (a) A wireframe view and (b) the system in practice.

Ueta T. et al. (2009) developed a prototype of a robotic surgical system to perform vitreoretinal surgery, which is illustrated in Fig. 3.5. They compared the average maximal deviation from the aiming point to the actual position of the tip of the instrument between manually conducted and robot-assisted surgeries. They concluded that the pointing accuracy was superior with the help of a robot, both on graph paper and in animal eye models.

Mitchell et al. (2007) developed and tested a new version of the steady hand manipulator (Fig. 3.6) introduced by Iordachita et al. (2006). The steady hand manipulator is used to perform retinal microsurgery and is illustrated in the following figure. In this system, the forces exerted by the surgeon on the tool are sensed, measured, and sent to a robotic controller. This robotic controller uses the received data in various control modes and provides smooth, tremor-free, precise positional control and force scaling.

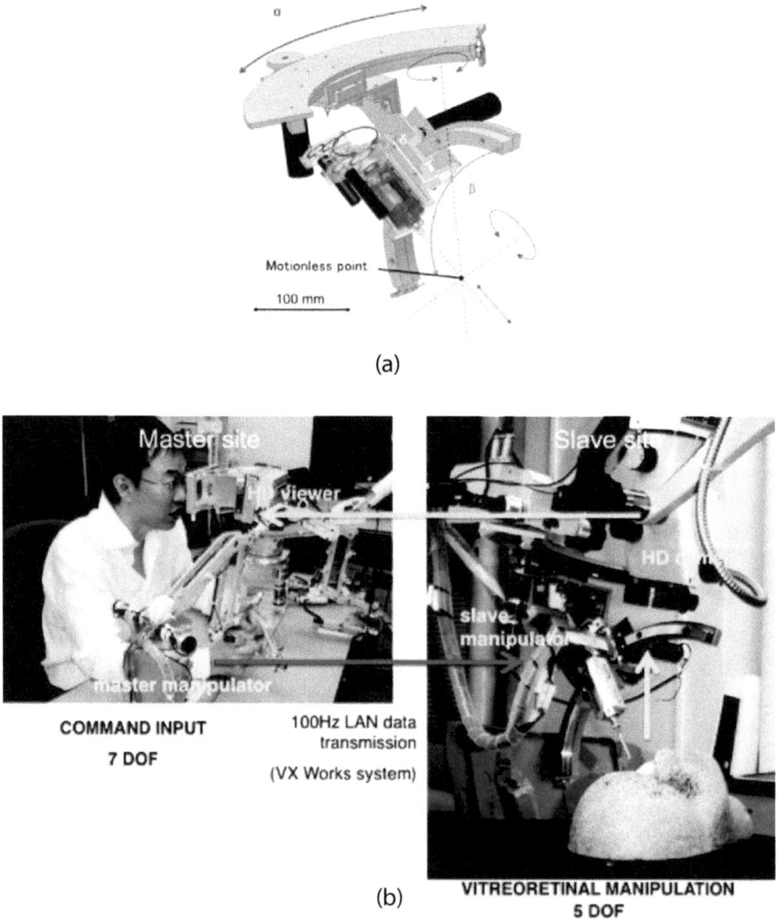


**Figure 3.5** Robotic system developed by Ueta et al. (2009). (a) The system parameters and (b) the system in practice.

Bourla et al. (2008) studied feasibility of intraocular robotic surgery with the da Vinci® Surgical System. They concluded that:

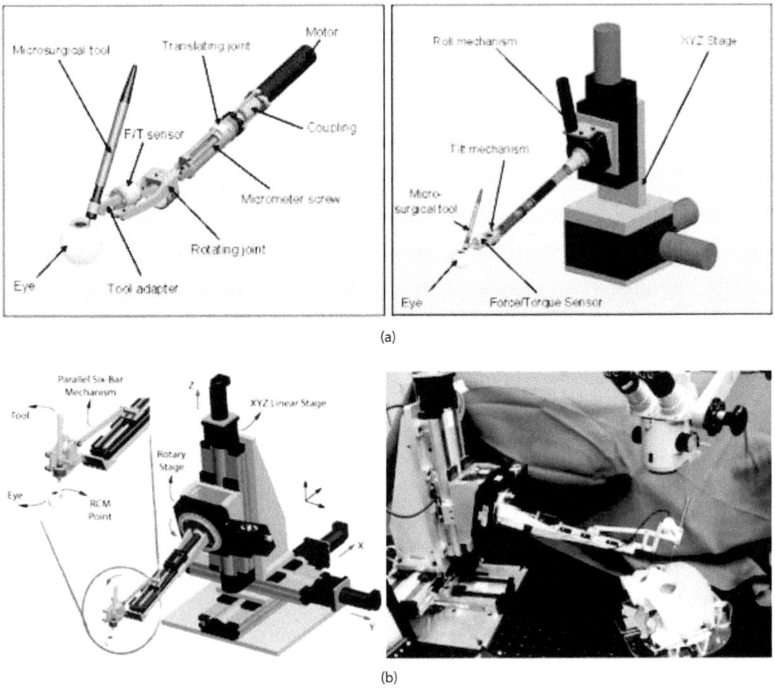


**Figure 3.6** Steady hand manipulator developed by Mitchell et al. (2007); different representations.

- the da Vinci® Surgical System has adequate dexterity to perform delicate intraocular manipulation
- the kinematics of the robotic arms is insufficient for standard intraocular surgery
- the system's endoscope did not provide as much detail as acquired by an ophthalmic microscope

Tsui et al. (2010) also further discuss the potential of the da Vinci® robot for ophthalmic surgery. They state that the da Vinci® robot is not an efficient system to use for intraocular surgery (Fig. 3.7) since the end-effector articulations start from a pivot point far from the tissue of interest and the end effectors are big relative to the application. These newer evaluations are opposing the result of (Tsirbas et al., 2007) which considered da Vinci surgical system a viable option for microsurgery.

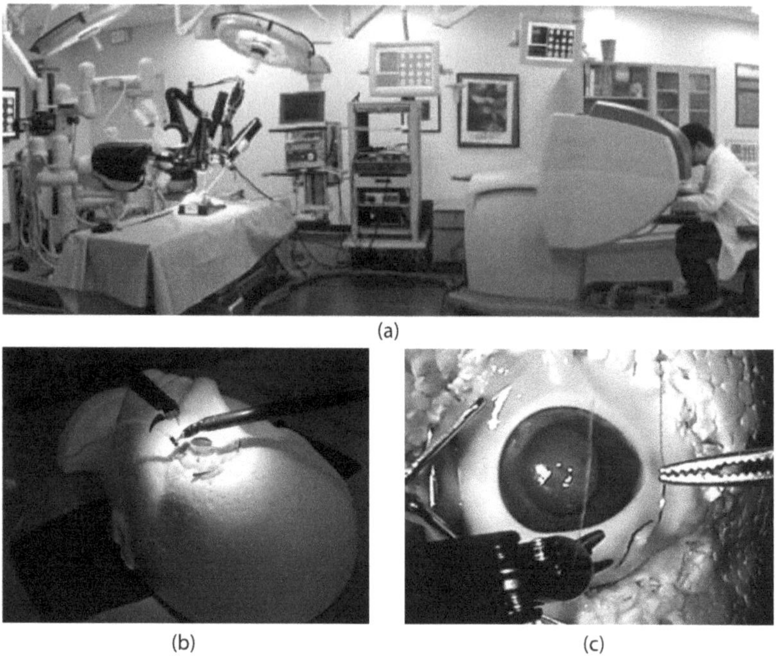

**Figure 3.7** Intraocular robotic surgery with the da Vinci® Surgical System.

# 3.3 Proposed Robotic Surgical System for Use in Ophthalmology

## 3.3.1 Introduction to Our System

The authors' experience and observations of ophthalmic surgeries at New York Eye and Ear Infirmity in the winter of 2011 while scrubbing with microsurgeon Dr. David Soltanpour disclosed an important characteristic of mechanical movements of surgical instruments and surgeons' hands in intraocular operations. This feature, which is the core idea behind the proposed robotic system, was that all surgical instruments in ophthalmic surgeries are inserted into the eye from its periphery. Accordingly, a ring-shaped surgical headmaster was considered in the proposed surgical system to be placed on top of the patient's head. Two or more robotic manipulators rotate around the surgical headmaster to deliver the surgical instruments from the periphery of the eye. The proposed robotic system is composed of two fundamental units, a master surgeon console/station and a robotic surgical slave (Figs. 3.8 and 3.9) (Shahinpoor et al. 2012). We discuss each next.

- *Master surgeon console.* The surgeon's station consists of an ergonomically-designed chair, a pair of vision goggles, and a pair of multiple-degrees-of-freedom joysticks. The joysticks can be installed on the chair with the help of two platforms. The imaging goggles generate a panoramic view of the surgical scene and assist the microsurgeon to maintain a natural posture and handle surgeries more easily and comfortably.

  Imaging features such as magnification further help the microsurgeon operate more precisely. The physician sits on the chair as the master of the robotic surgical procedure and controls the surgical operation via the joysticks. His/her hand movements are scaled, filtered, and translated into movements of surgical instruments snapped onto the robotic slave arms. Using a pair of joysticks and a pair of vision goggles is a space-efficient alternative to the current bulky surgeon stations.
- *Robotic surgical slave.* The surgical slave robot that actually performs the surgery on a patient's eye is illustrated in Fig. 3.8. It is composed of five main entities: a pedestal, a telescopic tower, the surgical headmaster, robotic arms, and an instrument holder. The pedestal is vibration-isolated, which can be securely locked in place. It moves the telescopic tower horizontally, to the left and right, to place the surgical headmaster above the right eye. The telescopic tower moves the surgical headmaster vertically up and down to position it at an appropriate height with respect to the patient's head.

  The surgical headmaster can also be moved horizontally in a telescopic manner, to the front and back, for further adjustment in the horizontal plane. It is placed at the right position in an *xyz* telescopic fashion. The headmaster is composed of an assembly of cylindrical precision head gears to which a fixed camera, a movable camera, and two or more movable precision multiple-axis robotic manipulators are attached. The fixed camera provides a top view of the surgical operation, while the movable camera rotates around the surgical headmaster to provide a peripheral view of the surgery. The movable camera is attached to a linear actuator, which can adjust its height.

  A rotary joint also changes its view angle. The two or more robotic manipulators revolve around the surgical headmaster to deliver precision surgical instruments from the periphery of the eye. Each robotic manipulator includes six main units: the base of the arm, a linear actuator in the base of the arm, a base rotary joint, an upper linear actuator, an elbow rotary joint, and a lower linear actuator. The base of the arm rotates the arms around the surgical headmaster. The linear actuator in the base of the arm moves the robotic arms in the radial direction. The base rotary joint rotates the robotic manipulator around the upper linear actuator's vertical axis. The upper linear actuator and lower linear actuator change their length to manipulate surgical instruments. The elbow rotary joint adjusts the angle between the upper linear actuator and the lower linear actuator.

The instrument holder holds the surgical instrument necessary in an operation for the robotic manipulators to pick them up. The instrument holder is in the workspace of the slave robot, and the robotic arms can easily pick any of the surgical instruments. The robotic end effectors are equipped with haptic feedback sensors, force sensors, and optical sensors, which help detect forces or disturbances experienced by the robotic end effectors by engaging with the eye anatomical parts.

All robotic movements and operations of the manipulator arms, end effectors, headmaster, and cameras are controlled by the master surgeon from the first major unit, the surgical master station.

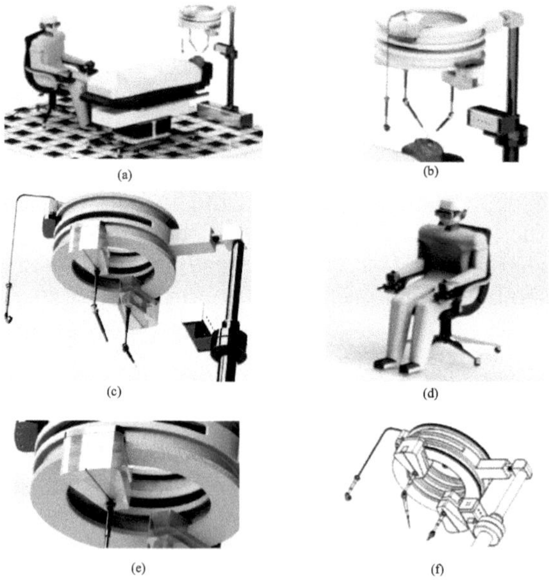

**Figure 3.8** The proposed robotic system for use in ophthalmic surgeries; different views.

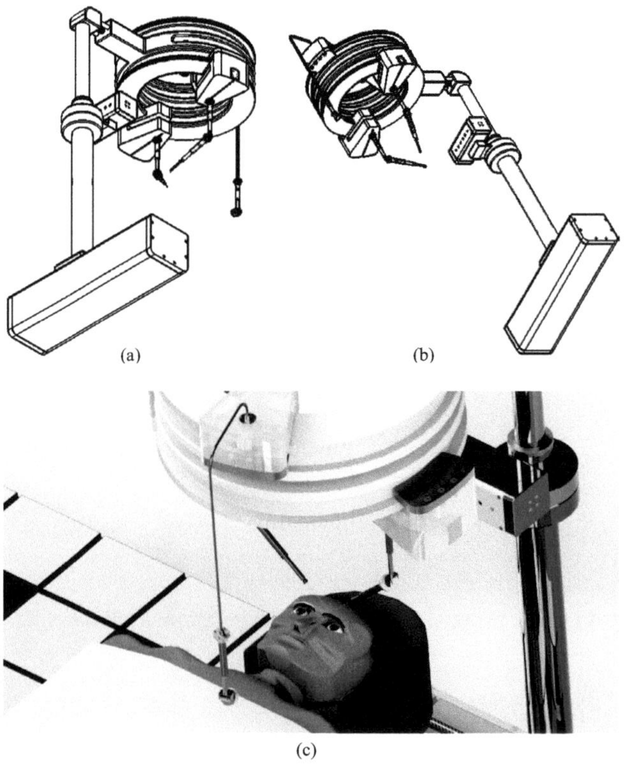


**Figure 3.9** The proposed robotic system for use in ophthalmic surgeries.

The following pictures (Fig. 3.10a,b) show the degrees of freedom of the proposed robotic system.

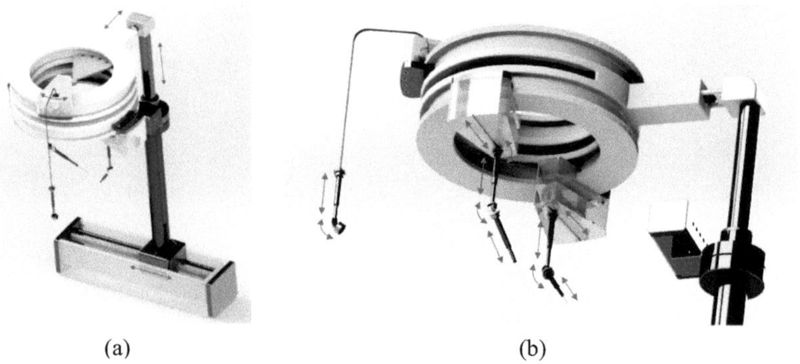


**Figure 3.10** Degrees of freedom of the proposed surgical system.

In the proposed surgical system (Figs. 3.11 and 3.12), at least one degree of rotational freedom is considered for surgical instruments. This rotation is about the axis of the lower linear actuators of the robotic arms, and its associated actuator is installed on the instrument itself.

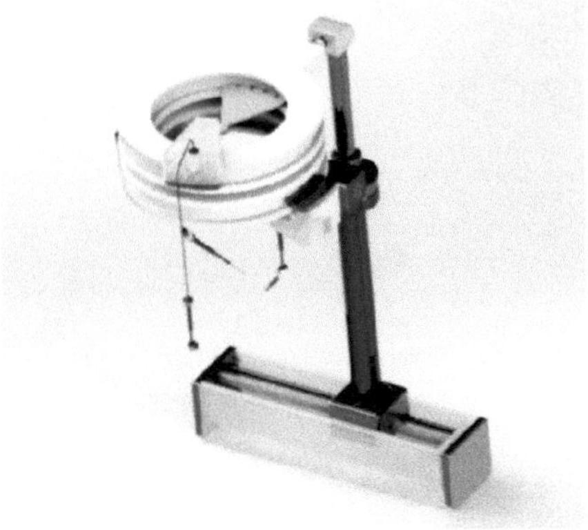

**Figure 3.11** The proposed robotic surgical system; a solid model.

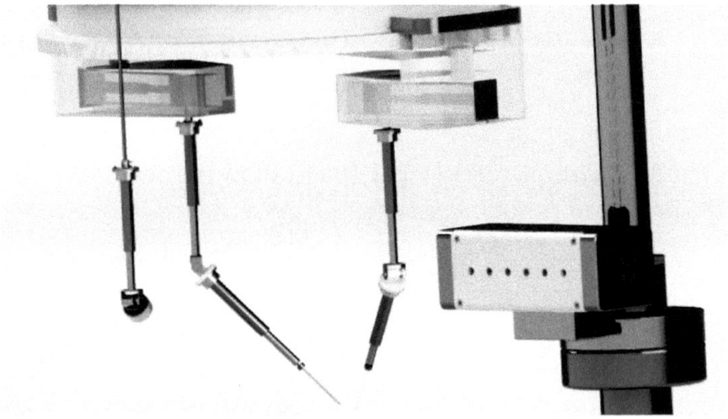

**Figure 3.12** The proposed robotic surgical system; a closer view of the robotic manipulators.

The proposed robotic surgical system can also be used for training medical students/residents (Figs. 3.13–3.16).
Different actuation methods and mechanisms can be utilized for altering the vector of joint parameters of the proposed system. These

methods include mechanical, hydraulic, pneumatic, piezoelectric, and electromagnetomechanical actuation, artificial muscles, and the use of parallel mechanisms.

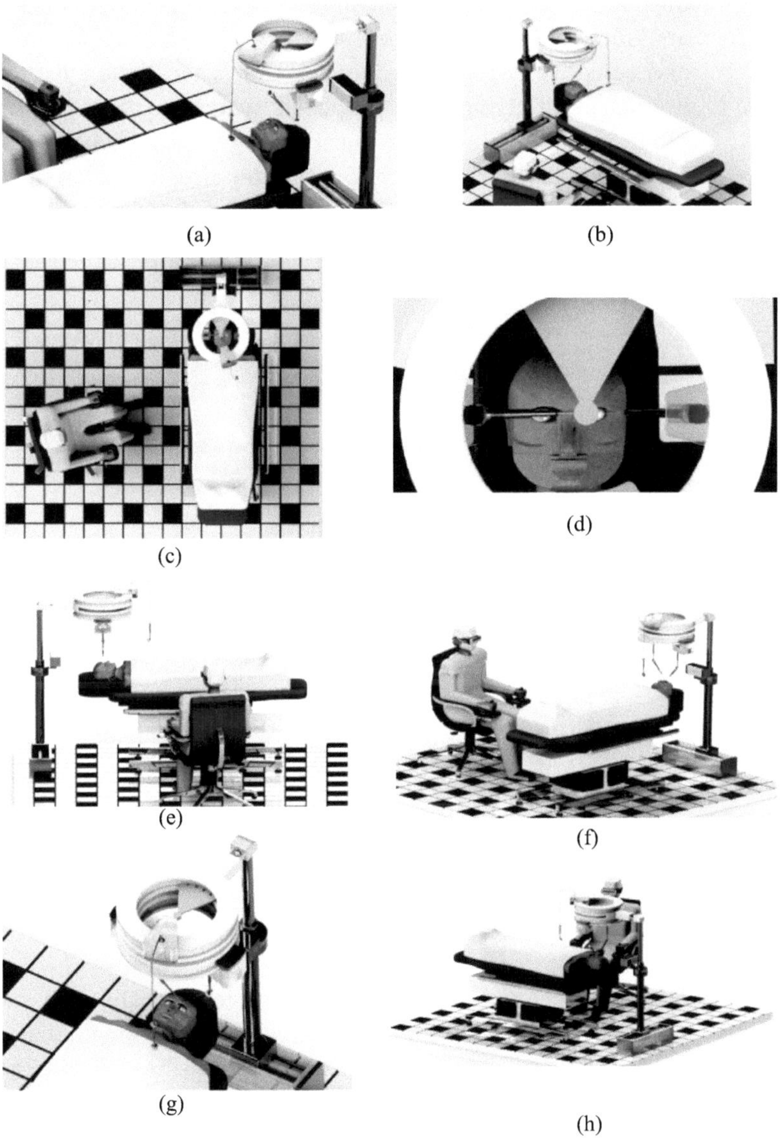


**Figure 3.13** Typical surgical scenes employing the proposed robotic surgical system.

Some features to be incorporated in this robotic system are as follows:

- *Hand tremor cancellation.* Movements of the surgeon's hands include natural tremor, which is inevitable. This is considered an issue when operating on the eye, because it is such a small and sensitive organ. The hand tremor cancellation feature is incorporated into the proposed system to increase the accuracy and decrease the uncertainty of the surgeon's hand movements. Thus, through a computer program, the shaky movements of the surgeon's hands are translated into smooth and tremor-free movements of the robotic manipulators.

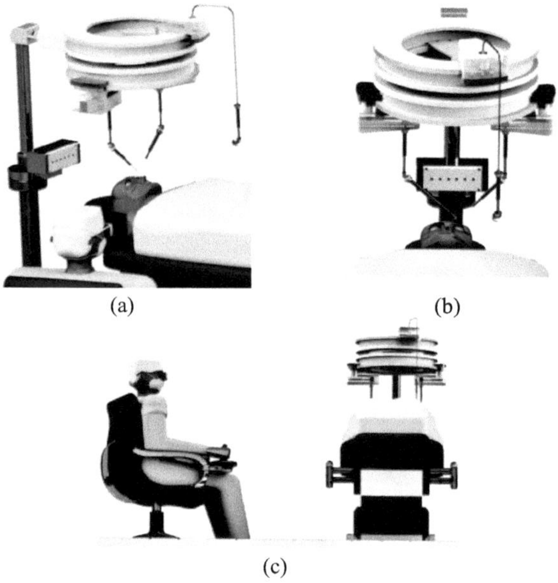

**Figure 3.14** Typical surgical scenes employing the proposed robotic surgical system.

- *Hand movement scaling.* Microsurgeries on the eye are performed through small incisions due to the small size of the target organ. For instance, in phacoemulsification cataract removal, surgery is performed through 2–3 mm incisions, and a scaling factor of less than 1, for example, 0.3, enables the surgeon to manipulate the surgical instruments with more precision and confidence. The scaling factor feature is incorporated in the proposed surgical system to increase the surgeon's maneuverability power.

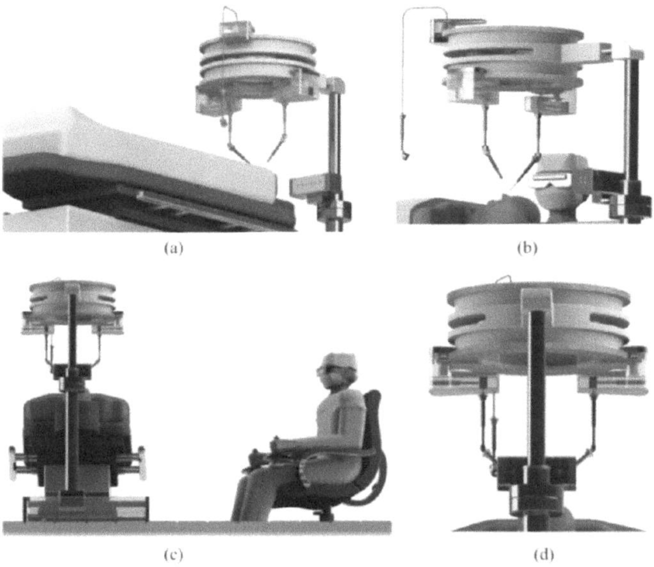


**Figure 3.15** Typical surgical scenes employing the proposed robotic surgical system.

- *Magnified vision.* This robotic system is equipped with a magnification feature, which provides the surgeon with a highly detailed representation of the surgical scene. The magnified vision assists the surgeon with making more precise movements.
- *Safety features.* Redundant safety features can be considered for this system in order to prevent any possible damage to the target organ. These features include position limit, speed limit, force limit, etc. These features prevent any sudden uncontrolled movement of the robotic manipulators.
- *Existence of a locking system.* In some cases, surgical instruments need to be held at a specific position and orientation for a while. For instance, in phacoemulsification cataract removal, if the cataract is hard the surgeon holds the probe in the same configuration until it breaks the hardened lens. The proposed system is equipped with a locking mechanism to keep both the joysticks and the robotic manipulators on hold, when necessary.

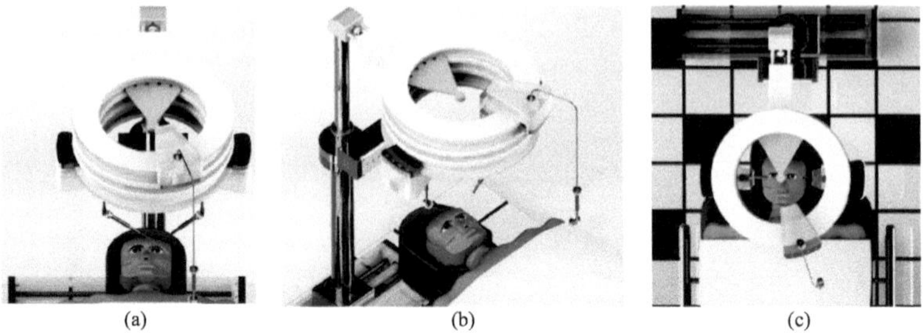

Figure 3.16 Typical surgical scenes employing the proposed robotic surgical system.

## 3.3.2 Forward and Inverse Kinematic Analysis

The Denavit–Hartenberg (D–H) transformation method is used to derive forward kinematics equations of the proposed surgical system. D–H coordinate systems and parameters are shown in Figs. 3.17–3.19. $x_{10}y_{10}z_{10}$ is a redundant coordinate frame. It is considered to take into account the lengths of the lower linear actuators and surgical instruments in the kinematic behavior of the system.

Table 3.1 shows the parameters of D–H method, specific to the intraocular robotic surgical system.

**Table 3.1** D–H parameters specific to the proposed intraocular robotic surgical system

| D–H coordinate frame | $\theta_i$ | $\alpha_i$ | $a_i$ | $d_i$ |
|---|---|---|---|---|
| 1 | 0 | 0 | 0 | 0 |
| 2 | 270 | 270 | 0 | $d_2$ |
| 3 | 90 | 270 | 0 | $d_3$ |
| 4 | 0 | 90 | 0 | $d_4$ |
| 5 | $\theta_5$ | 90 | 0 | 0 |
| 6 | 0 | 90 | 0 | $R - r$ |
| 7 | $-\theta_7$ | 0 | 0 | 0 |
| 8 | 90 | 90 | 0 | $d_8$ |
| 9 | $\theta_9$ | 270 | 0 | 0 |
| 10 | 0 | 0 | 0 | $d_{10}$ |

Then the relative transformation matrix of the D–H coordinate systems $i - 1$ and $i$ can be calculated using Eq. 2.11:

$$A_{i-1}^{i} = A_i = \begin{bmatrix} \cos\theta_i & -\cos\alpha_i \cdot \sin\theta_i & \sin\alpha_i \cdot \sin\theta_i & a_i \cdot \cos\theta_i \\ \sin\theta_i & \cos\alpha_i \cdot \cos\theta_i & -\sin\alpha_i \cdot \cos\theta_i & a_i \cdot \sin\theta_i \\ 0 & \sin\alpha_i & \cos\alpha_i & di \\ 0 & 0 & 0 & 1 \end{bmatrix}$$

We have

$$A_1 = \begin{bmatrix} 1 & 0 & 0 & 0 \\ 0 & 1 & 0 & 0 \\ 0 & 0 & 1 & 0 \\ 0 & 0 & 0 & 1 \end{bmatrix}; A_2 = \begin{bmatrix} 0 & 0 & 1 & 0 \\ -1 & 0 & 0 & 0 \\ 0 & -1 & 0 & d_2 \\ 0 & 0 & 0 & 1 \end{bmatrix}; A_3 = \begin{bmatrix} 0 & 0 & -1 & 0 \\ 1 & 0 & 0 & 0 \\ 0 & -1 & 0 & d_3 \\ 0 & 0 & 0 & 1 \end{bmatrix};$$

$$A_4 = \begin{bmatrix} 1 & 0 & 0 & 0 \\ 0 & 0 & -1 & 0 \\ 0 & 1 & 0 & d_4 \\ 0 & 0 & 0 & 1 \end{bmatrix}$$

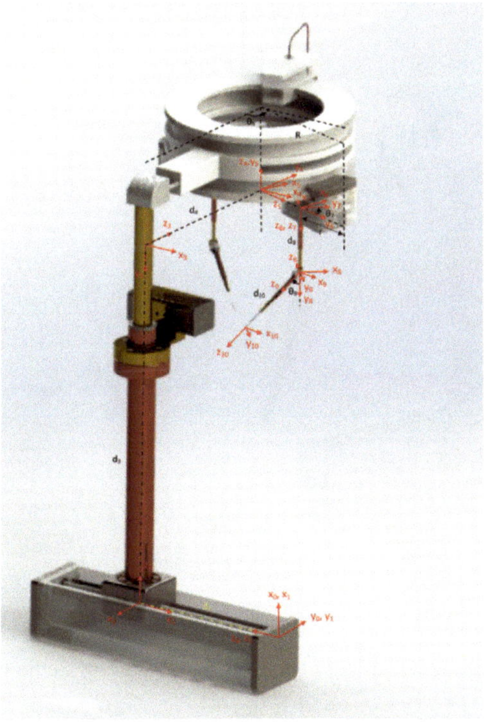

**Figure 3.17** D–H coordinate systems on the proposed robotic surgical system.

$$A_5 = \begin{bmatrix} \cos\theta_5 & 0 & \sin\theta_5 & 0 \\ \sin\theta_5 & 0 & -\cos\theta_5 & 0 \\ 0 & 1 & 0 & 0 \\ 0 & 0 & 0 & 1 \end{bmatrix}; A_6 = \begin{bmatrix} 1 & 0 & 0 & 0 \\ 0 & 0 & -1 & 0 \\ 0 & 1 & 0 & R-r \\ 0 & 0 & 0 & 1 \end{bmatrix};$$

$$A_7 = \begin{bmatrix} \cos\theta_7 & \sin\theta_7 & 0 & 0 \\ -\sin\theta_7 & \cos\theta_7 & 0 & 0 \\ 0 & 0 & 1 & 0 \\ 0 & 0 & 0 & 1 \end{bmatrix}$$

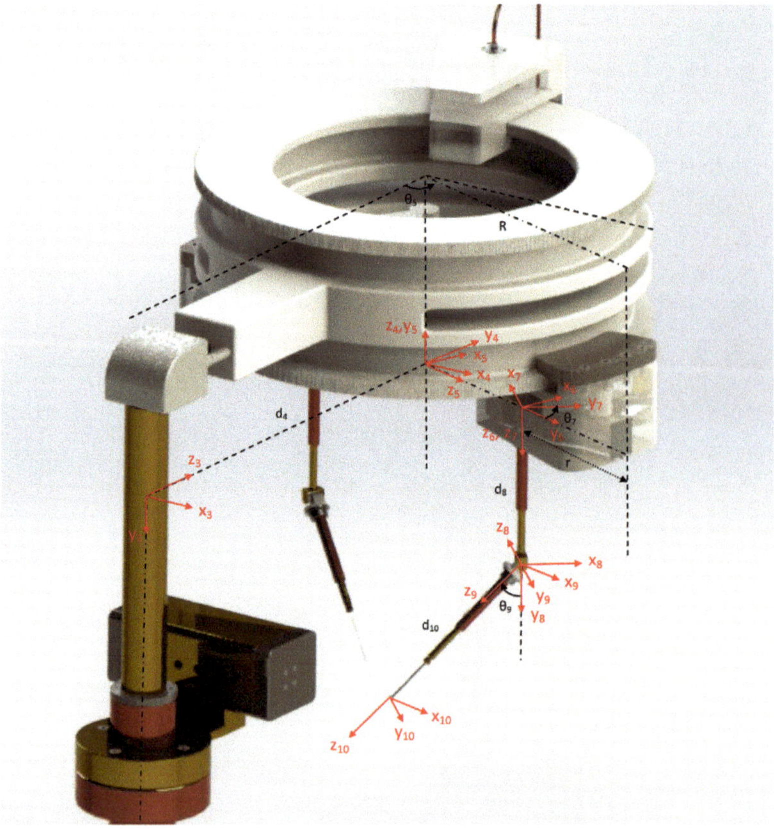


**Figure 3.18** A closer view of the D–H coordinate systems on the proposed system.

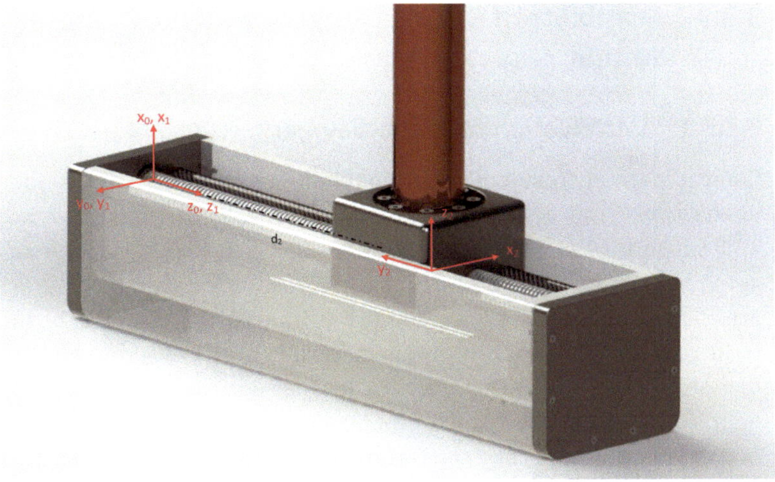


**Figure 3.19** A closer view of the D–H coordinate systems on the proposed system.

$$A_8 = \begin{bmatrix} 0 & 0 & 1 & 0 \\ 1 & 0 & 0 & 0 \\ 0 & 1 & 0 & d_8 \\ 0 & 0 & 0 & 1 \end{bmatrix}; A_9 = \begin{bmatrix} \cos\theta_9 & 0 & -\sin\theta_9 & 0 \\ \sin\theta_9 & 0 & \cos\theta_9 & 0 \\ 0 & -1 & 0 & 0 \\ 0 & 0 & 0 & 1 \end{bmatrix};$$

$$A_{10} = \begin{bmatrix} 1 & 0 & 0 & 0 \\ 0 & 1 & 0 & 0 \\ 0 & 0 & 1 & d_{10} \\ 0 & 0 & 0 & 1 \end{bmatrix}$$

According to Eq. 2.9 we can easily obtain the D–H transformation matrix of the proposed surgical system by multiplying the ten calculated **A**s.

$$\mathbf{T_n} = \mathbf{A}_1 \cdot \mathbf{A}_2 \cdot \mathbf{A}_3 \cdot \mathbf{A}_4 \cdot \mathbf{A}_5 \cdot \mathbf{A}_6 \cdot \mathbf{A}_7 \cdot \mathbf{A}_8 \cdot \mathbf{A}_9 \cdot \mathbf{A}_{10} \qquad (3.1)$$

Advanced numerical methods can be used to analyze inverse kinematics of the proposed robotic system since there is no interest in pursuing an analytical solution for such complex forward kinematics equations. Inverse kinematics analysis is not covered in this book.

## 3.3.3 Feasibility of Cataract Surgery with the Proposed System

### 3.3.3.1 Introduction to cataract surgery

Cataracts are the result of metabolic changes in crystalline lens fibers of the eyes—more specifically, denaturation of the lens protein—and cause loss of visual acuity and contrast sensitivity. Although aging is a typical cause of development of cataracts and cataracts are common among elderly people, they may also occur by exposure to ultraviolet light, entry of toxic materials in the eye, diseases like diabetes, congenital defects, etc. An eye lens with a cataract disperses light and causes poor focus of images on the retina. This results in blurry vision. A report by the National Eye Institute states that about half of the US population that is 65 years old or more has cataracts. Figure 3.20a depicts a normal eye with a clear lens, and Fig. 3.20b depicts an eye with a cataractous lens.

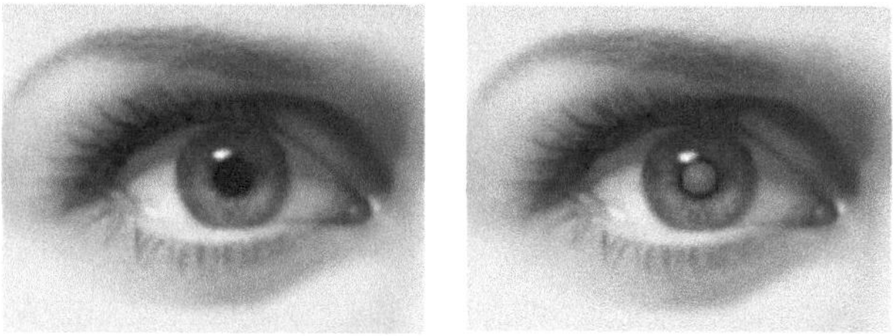

(a) (b)

**Figure 3.20** Eye with (a) a clear lens and (b) a cataractous lens.[3]

There are both nonsurgical and surgical methods to treat cataracts. Nonsurgical methods suggest application of eyedrops if the cataract is not fully developed. However, fully developed cataracts imply surgical treatments during which the natural lens of the eye is removed and replaced with an artificial IOL. More than 1.5 million cataract surgeries are performed in the United States each year, which makes cataract surgery the most common ophthalmic surgery.

There are three types of cataract surgery: phacoemulsification, extracapsular cataract extraction (ECCE), and intracapsular cataract

[3]http://www.mynewyorkeyedoctor.com/uncategorized/i-was-told-i-have-a-cataract-what-should-i-do

extraction (ICCE). Phacoemulsification is performed through 2–3 mm incisions and hence is minimally invasive. This type of intraocular surgery is common in developed countries. Short surgery time and quick recovery make this method popular. However, ECCE is widely used in developing countries due to the high cost of phacoemulsification cataract surgery. ICCE is an outdated method and is rarely used. The appropriate type of cataract surgery is determined by microsurgeons, depending on the amount of cataract development, the patient's condition, cost, etc. In the following section, we describe phacoemulsification cataract surgery in detail and discuss the feasibility of doing this type of operation by the proposed robotic system.

#### 3.3.3.2 Phacoemulsification with the proposed robotic system

All steps in performing a phacoemulsification cataract surgery are described here:

1. *Anesthesia and pupil dilation.* Cataract surgery usually involves administration of local anesthetic eyedrops or numbing eyedrops such as Minims amethocaine, in addition to systemic sedation administered by an anesthesiologist or nurse anesthetist. Anesthesia may be placed topically (eyedrops) or via injection next to (peribulbar) or behind (retrobulbar) the eye (Fig. 3.21). Dilation of the pupil is followed, as shown in Fig. 3.22.

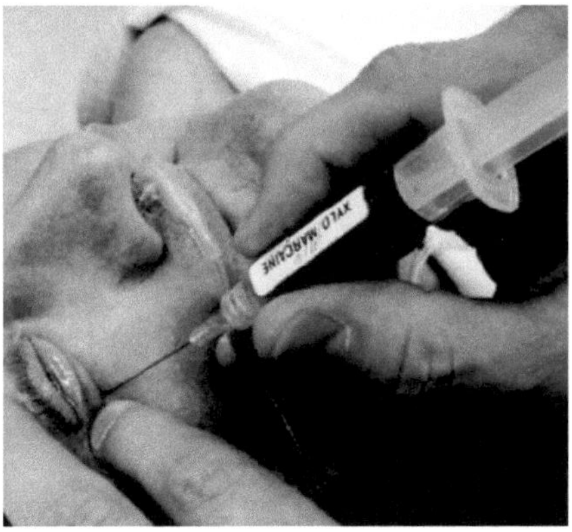

**Figure 3.21** Retrobulbar anesthesia.[4]

[4]http://webeye.ophth.uiowa.edu/eyeforum/atlas/pages/retrobulbar-block-before-cataract-surgery.html

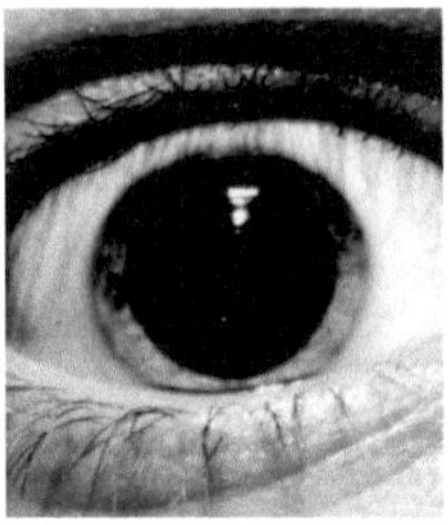

**Figure 3.22** Dilated pupil.[5]

Figure 3.23 shows the ability of the proposed robotic surgical system to give anesthetic injection to different parts of the eye.

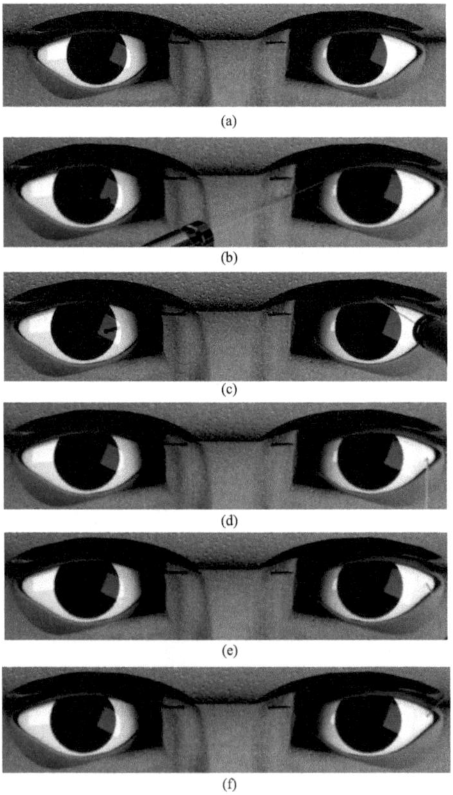


**Figure 3.23** Anesthetic injection to different parts of the eye by the proposed robotic system.

[5]http://mediqbank.blogspot.com/2010/05/neurology-mcqpart-04.html

The pupil is then dilated using drops to help better visualize the cataract by the camera systems. Pupil-dilating eyedrops such as atropine are used. These steps are all done by an anesthesiologist or nurse anesthetist. General anesthesia is rarely necessary but may be employed for children and adults with particular medical or other relevant issues. The eyelids and surrounding skin will be swabbed with disinfectant by the robotic end effectors. The face is covered with a cloth or sheet, with an opening for the operative eye.

Figure 3.24 shows the ability of the proposed robotic surgical system to apply eyedrops to dilate the eye.

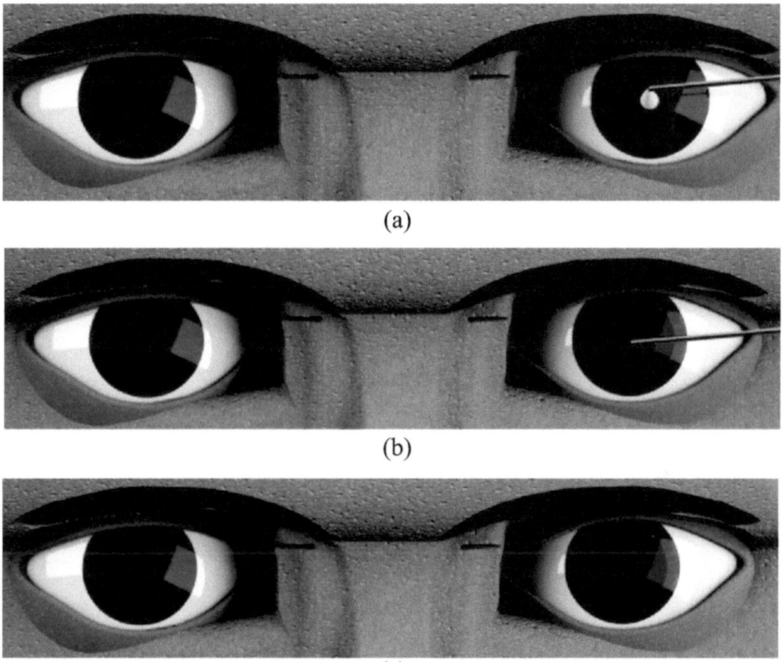

(a)

(b)

(c)

**Figure 3.24** Application of pupil-dilating eyedrops by the proposed robotic system.

2. *Exposure of the eyeball using a lid speculum.* The eyelid is held open by a nurse or a doctor with a speculum to minimize blinking during surgery (Fig. 3.25a,b).

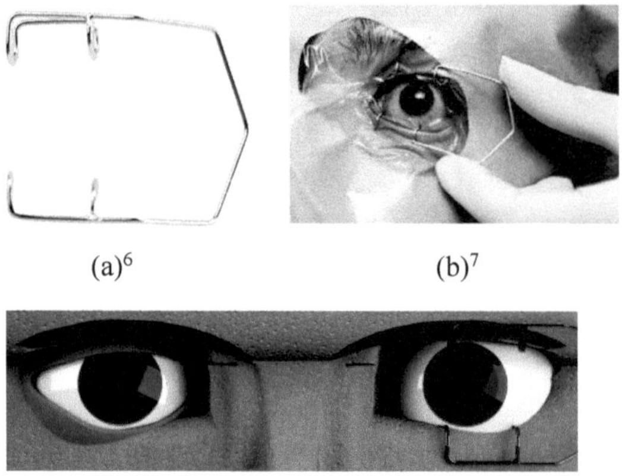

(a)[6] (b)[7]

(c)

**Figure 3.25** Application of an eyelid speculum: (a) a lid speculum, (b) the lid speculum in use, (c) a lid speculum on our model

3. *Paracentesis.* The purpose is to provide an entry port to the anterior chamber of the eye through the keratolimbal region of the eye to inject anesthetics and/or viscoelastic gel material to the anterior chamber. This paracentesis track (Fig. 3.26a,b) is then used to allow introduction of a second instrument (keratome) in the eye to perform capsulorhexis and phacoemulsification. The ocular surface is kept moist using sterile saline eyedrops or methylcellulose viscoelastic material.

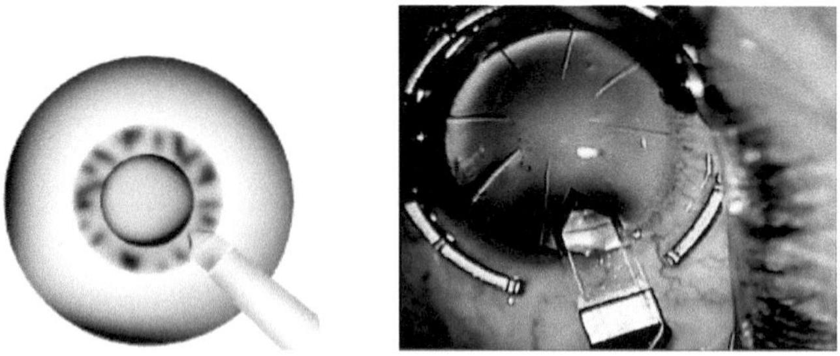

(a)[8] (b)[9]

**Figure 3.26** Paracentesis.

[6]http://www.wemed1.com/products/received.asp?offset=1600
[7]http://www.visionforum.co.uk/2011/03/lasik-eye-surgery/
[8]http://emedicine.medscape.com/article/1844198-technique (December 03, 2012)
[9]http://www.ophthalmologymanagement.com/articleviewer.aspx?articleid=102450

Figure 3.27a–d shows the ability of the proposed robotic surgical system to perform paracentesis.

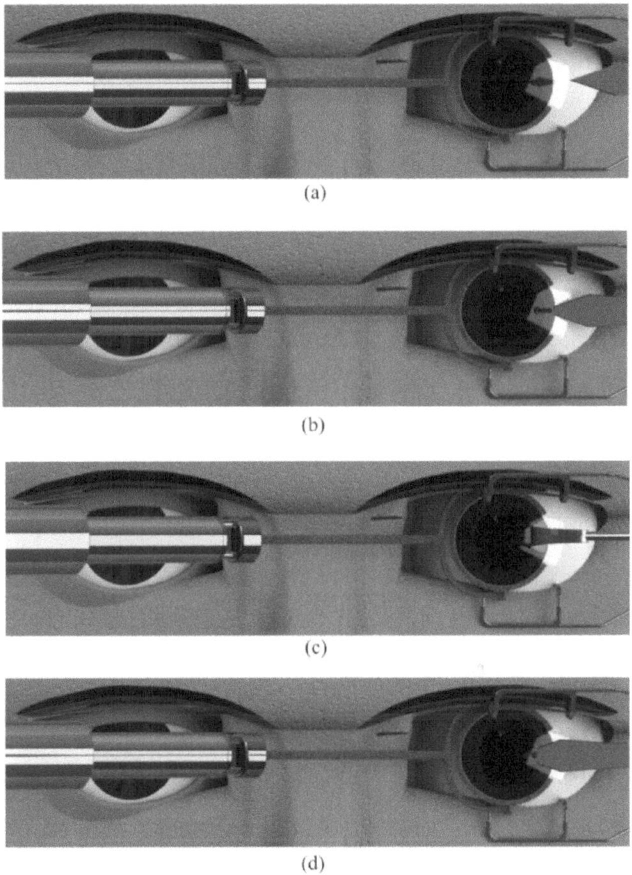


**Figure 3.27** The proposed robotic system performing paracentesis.

Viscoelastic gel injection is performed robotically to stabilize the anterior chamber and to help maintain the shape of the eye and cornea as well as pressurization of the eye, which prevents it from collapse during surgery (Fig. 3.28a,b). Sometimes during paracentesis the eye is stabilized with a Thornton fixation ring. This ring, or a modification thereof, provides tractional feet with which the globe may be stabilized. Some gentle downward pressure may be applied to maintain traction. Some microsurgeons use a cotton tip applicator, applied at the limbus with the dominant hand.

Some microsurgeons use 0.12 forceps either to grasp the sclera for stability or to straddle the site of entry to prevent eye rotation. These types of stabilization of the eye during cataract surgery will also be performed by robotic end effectors. Careful consideration is given to the proximity between the paracentesis channel and the main wound by keratome for capsulorhexis and phacoemulsification to prevent the instruments from tangling up (or locking), which makes manipulating instruments in the eye difficult. Thus the robotic system must typically space the paracentesis about 90 degrees away from the eventual main wound. The blades for creating a paracentesis vary, but the goal is to create a 1 mm wide incision. The robotic system must maintain blade positioning until the blade is completely removed from the eye in order to avoid undesirable widening of the wound from a misguided blade edge while exiting.

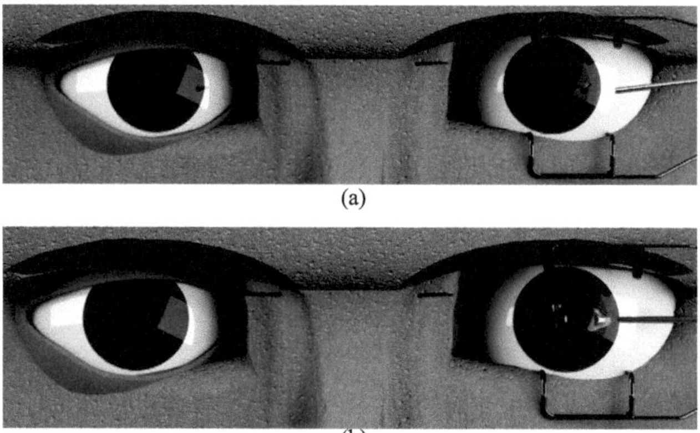

(a)

(b)

**Figure 3.28** The proposed robotic system injecting viscoelastic gel.

4. *Capsulorhexis.* Capsulorhexis is a procedure that includes a capsulotomy, rarely known as cystitomy, which consists of cutting open a portion of the lens capsule to access the lens inside (see Fig. 3.29a–d). An anterior capsulotomy refers to the opening of the front portion of the lens capsule, whereas a posterior capsulotomy refers to the opening of the back portion of the lens capsule. In phacoemulsification, the surgeon performs an anterior continuous curvilinear capsulorhexis to create a round and smooth opening through which the lens nucleus can be emulsified and the IOL implant inserted.

Specially designed capsulorhexis forceps are used to create a circular opening in anterior or posterior capsulorhexis.

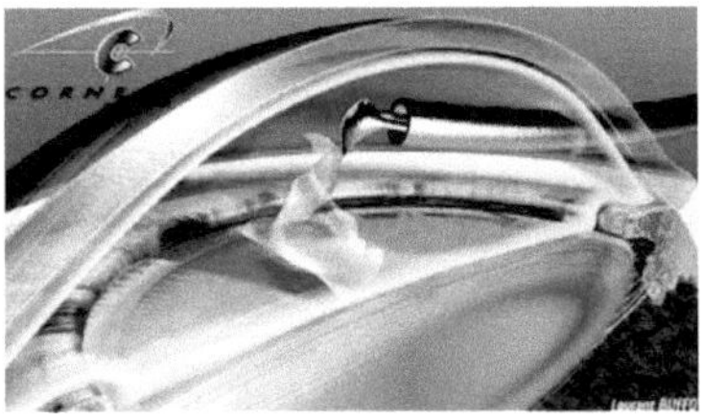

(c) [10]

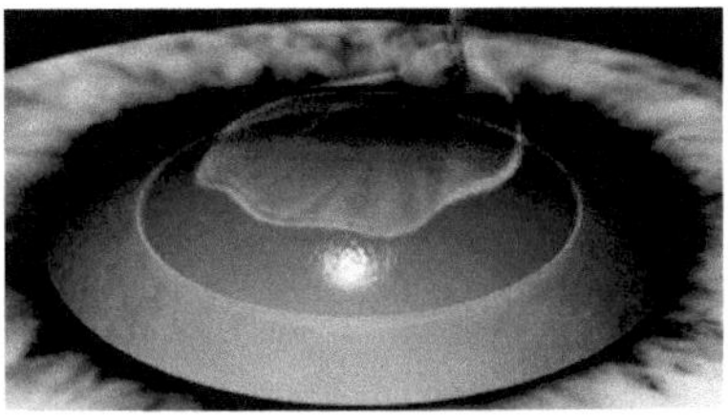

(d)[11]

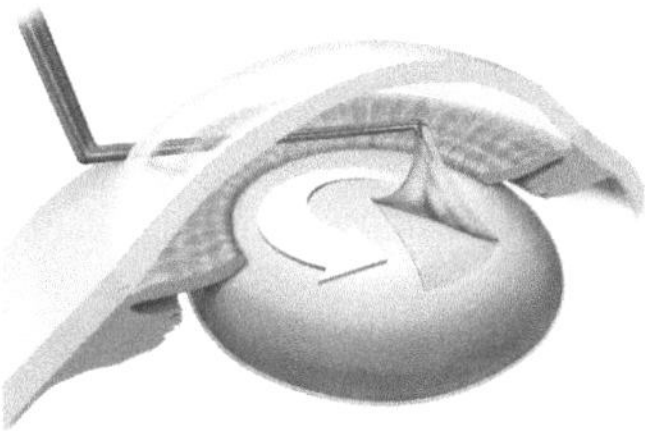

(c) [12]

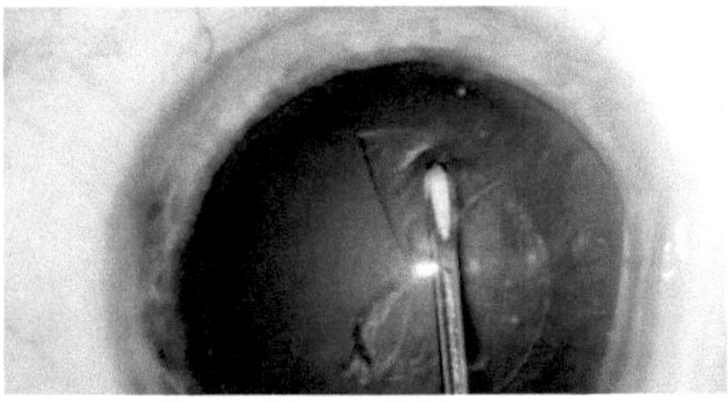

(d)[13]

**Figure 3.29** Capsulorhexis; different representations.

Figure 3.30a–e shows the ability of the proposed robotic surgical system to perform capsulorhexis.

5. *Hydrodissection and hydrodelineation.* Jets of special fluids are used through special cannulas to perform hydrodissection, which weakens the capsular–cortical connections and creates lens mobility during phacoemulsification (Fig. 3.31). Following hydrodissection, the surgeon performs hydrodelineation (Fig. 3.32) to separate the endonucleus and epinucleus (Fig. 3.33). These techniques are helpful in preventing posterior capsule tear during phacoemulsification. These procedures will also be performed by robotic end effectors under the supervision of the microsurgeon.

[10]http://phacobimanuelle.net/en/technique-capsulorhexis/
[11]http://www.josydoodle.com/breakdown.html
[12]http://luminaryvisuals.com/portfolio.html
[13]http://vimeo.com/26537200

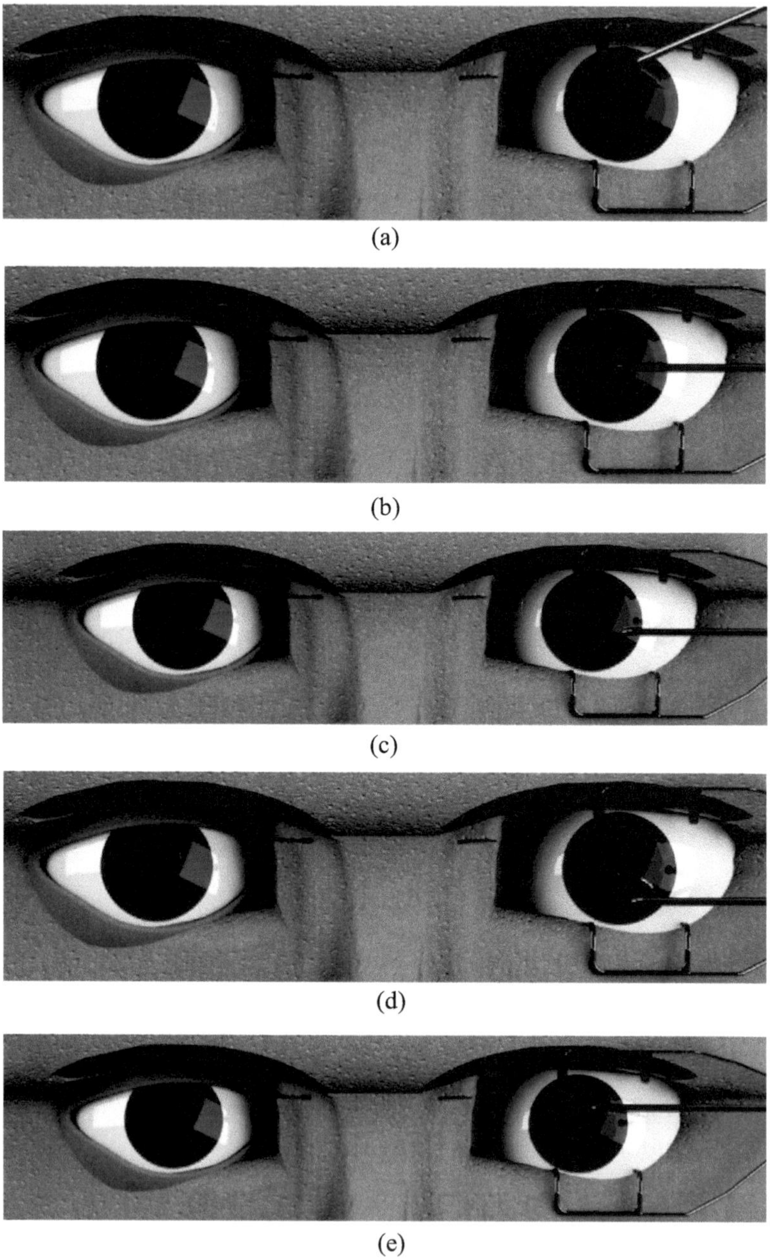


**Figure 3.30** The proposed robotic system performing capsulorhexis.

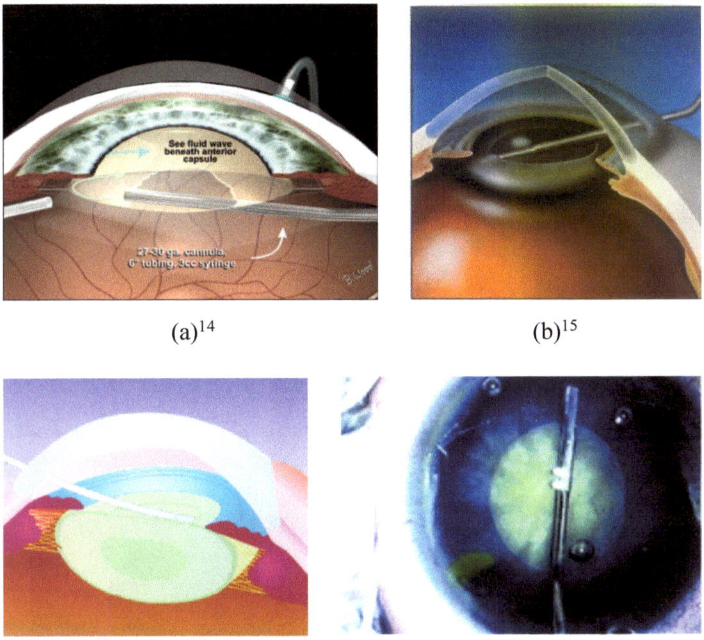


(a)[14] (b)[15]

(c)[16] (d)[17]

**Figure 3.31** Hydrodissection; different representations.

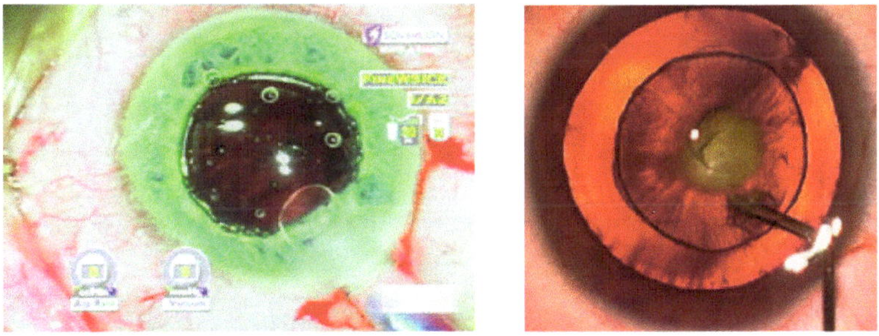

(a)[18] (b)[19]

**Figure 3.32** Hydrodelineation; different representations.

---

[14]http://www.retinalphysician.com/articleviewer.aspx?articleID=107237

[15]http://ocularis.es/blog/?p=39

[16]http://www.optech.net.au/Steriseal/hydrodissection.html

[17]http://www.eyeworld.org/article.php?sid=2325

[18]http://www.eyeworld.org/article.php?sid=3103

[19]http://www.eyeworld.org/printarticle.php?id=3910

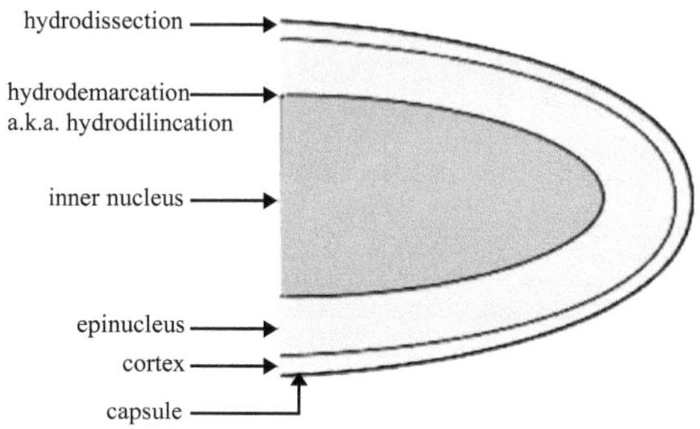


**Figure 3.33** Hydrodissection and hydrodelineation.[20]

Figure 3.34 shows the ability of the proposed robotic surgical system to perform hydrodissection or hydrodelineation.

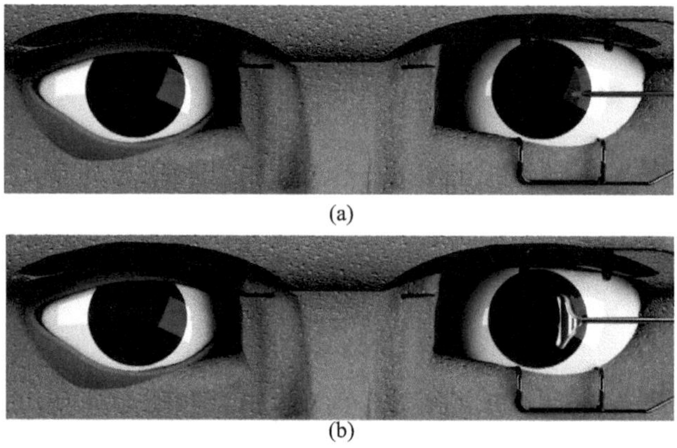


**Figure 3.34** The proposed robotic system performing (a) hydrodissection and (b) hydrodelineation.

6. *Phacoemulsification of the cataract lens.* The surgical procedure in phacoemulsification (Figs. 3.35–3.37) for removal of a cataract involves a number of steps, as described above, consisting of anesthesia, exposure using a lid speculum, entry into the eye through a minimal incision (corneal or scleral), viscoelastic injection to stabilize the anterior chamber, capsulorhexis, hydrodissection, and hydrodelineation. This

[20]http://www.cybersight.org/bins/content_page.asp?cid=735-2858-4398-11916-11902-11908

will be followed by ultrasonic emulsification of the cataract after nuclear cracking or chopping (if needed), cortical aspiration of the lens, and capsular polishing (if needed).

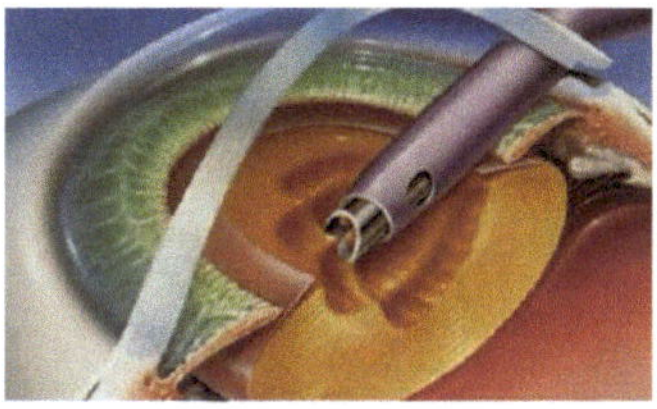

(a)[21]

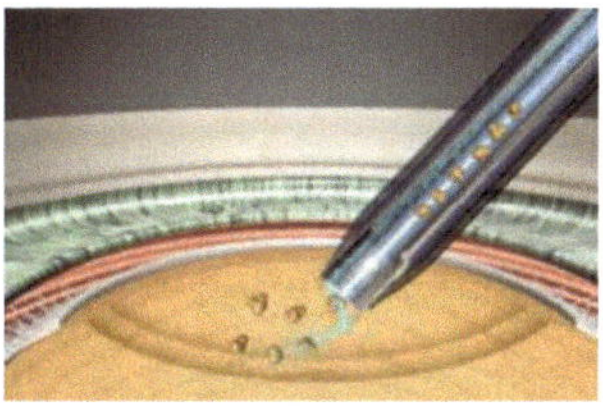

(b)[22]

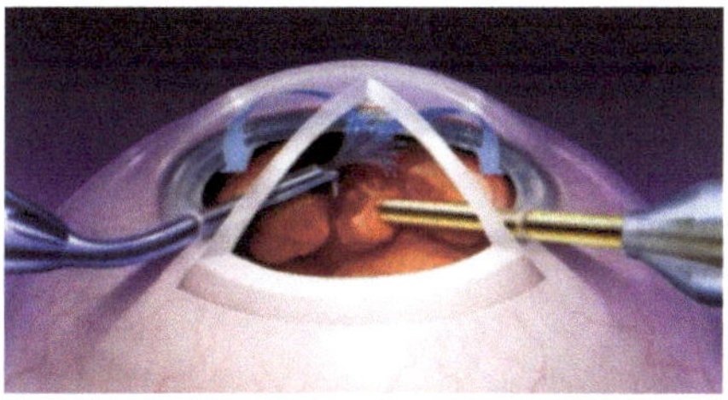

(c)[23]

**Figure 3.35** Phacoemulsification; different representations.

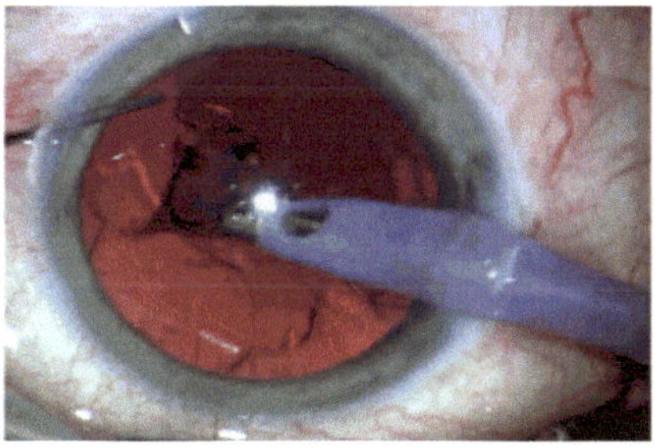

(a)[24]

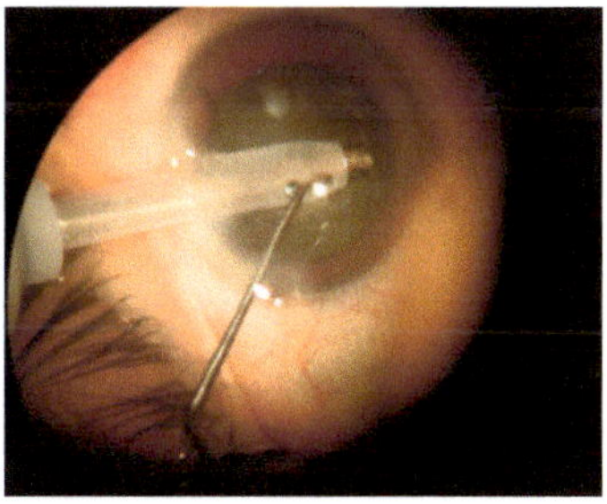

(b)[25]

**Figure 3.36** Phacoemulsification in practice.

---

[21]http://www.eyedoctor.com.tw/EN/cata5.aspx

[22]http://eastmichiganeyecenter.com/index.cfm/PageID/6919

[23]http://phacobimanuelle.net/fr/technique-nucleofracture/

[24]http://www.sightnation.com/news/phacoemulsification-related-endothelial-cell-loss-proves-higher-transplanted-corneas

[25]http://www.cataract-surgery-recovery.net/phacoemulsification-cataract-surgery.html

Figure 3.37 shows the ability of the proposed robotic surgical system to perform phacoemulsification.

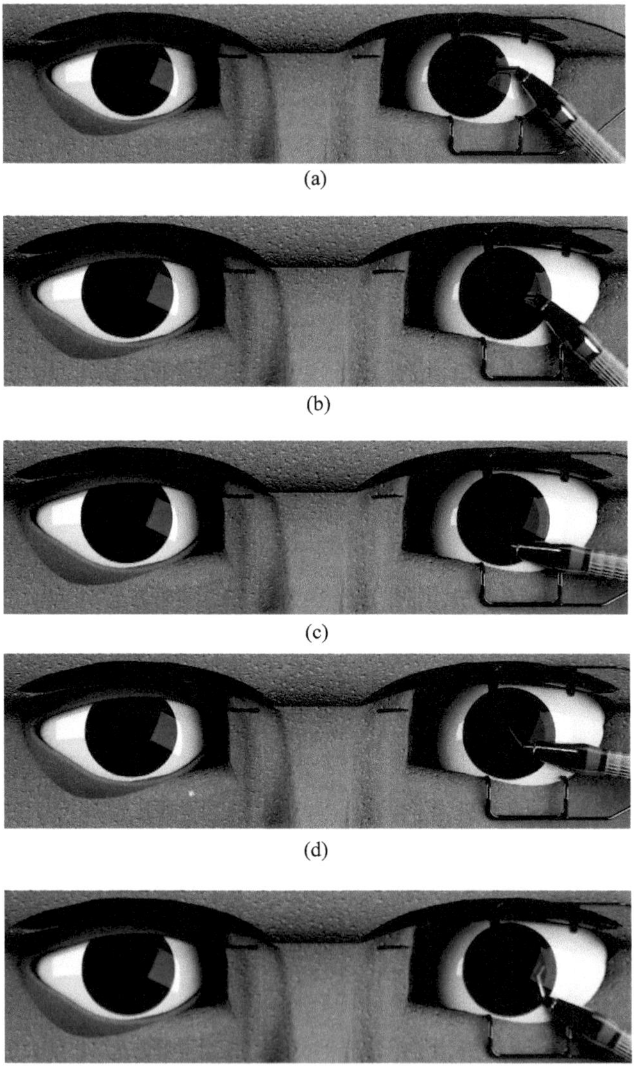


**Figure 3.37** The proposed robotic system performing phacoemulsification.

7. *Implantation of an artificial IOL.* Following cataract removal by phacoemulsification, an IOL (Figs. 3.38–3.41) is usually

inserted. After the IOL is inserted, the surgeon checks to ensure that the incision does not leak fluid. This is a very important step since wound leakage increases the risk of unwanted microorganisms gaining access into the eye and predisposes the patient to endophathalmitis. An antibiotic/steroid combination eyedrop is put, and an eye shield may be applied on the operated eye, sometimes supplemented with an eye patch.

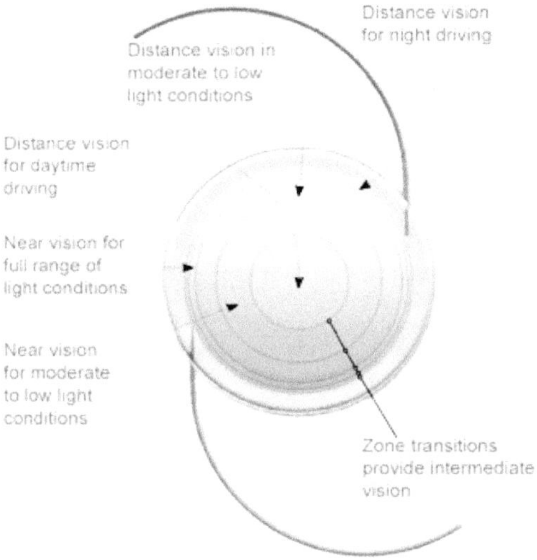


**Figure 3.38** The structure of a common artificial IOL.[26]

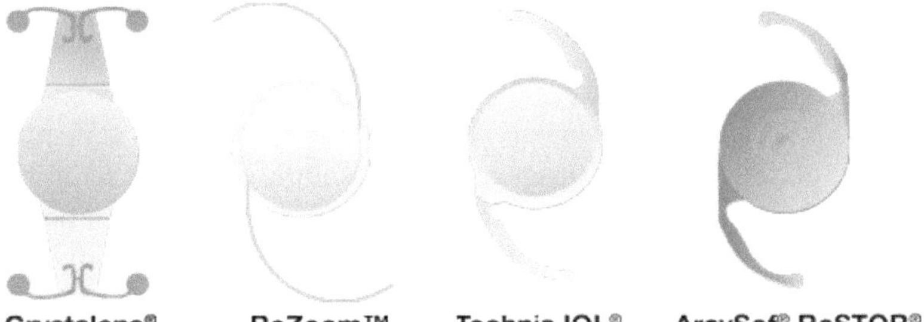


**Figure 3.39** Different commercial artificial IOLs.[27]

[26]http://www.tour2india4health.com/intra-ocular-lens-lmplant-surgery-india.htm
[27]http://www.jupitercataract.com/florida/cataract-center/premium-lens-implants.htm

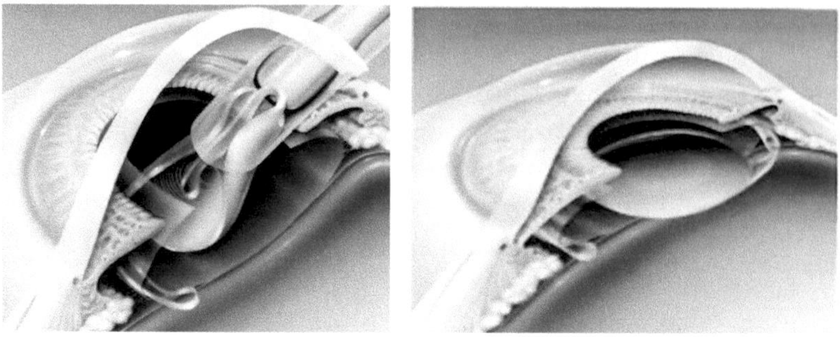

(a)[28] (b)[29]

**Figure 3.40** Implanting an artificial IOL.

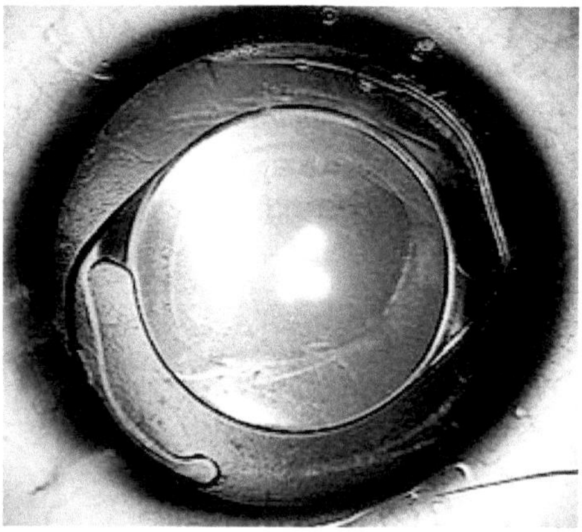

**Figure 3.41** An artificial IOL in place.[30]

Figure 3.42 shows the ability of the proposed robotic surgical system to implant an artificial IOL.

8. *Viscoelastic gel removal.* After the implantation and centration of the IOL, the viscoelastic gel should be drained out of the anterior chamber (Fig. 3.43). The one complication of viscoelastic materials is that they may cause postoperative IOP to rise. Thus, they need to be completely cleaned out. These viscoelastic materials may be sodium hyaluronate (Healon), Healon GV, chondroitin sulfatesodium hyaluronate (Viscoat),

[28]http://iollens.com/intraocular-lens-iol-2/

[29]http://www.silmakirurgia.ee/en/For-patient/Surgery/Multifocal-IOL

[30]http://www.aapos.org/terms/conditions/61

hydroxypropylmethylcellulose (Occucoat), polyacrylamide (Orcolon), and many more. Viscoelastic gels are normally aspirated using an automated irrigation/aspiration device.

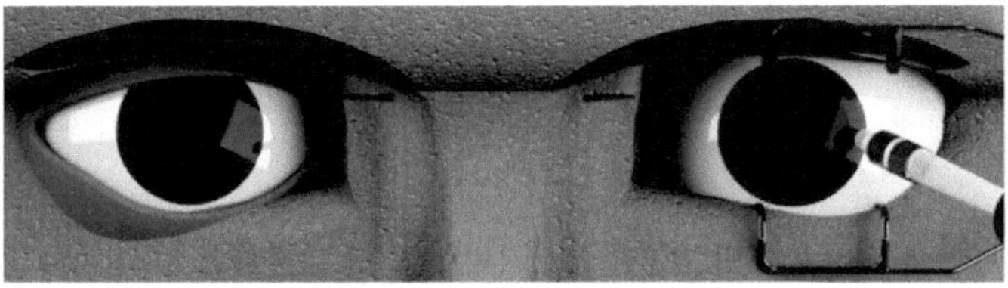

(a)

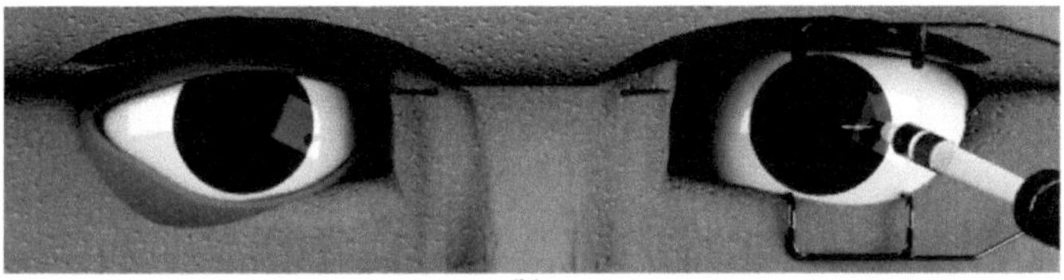

(b)

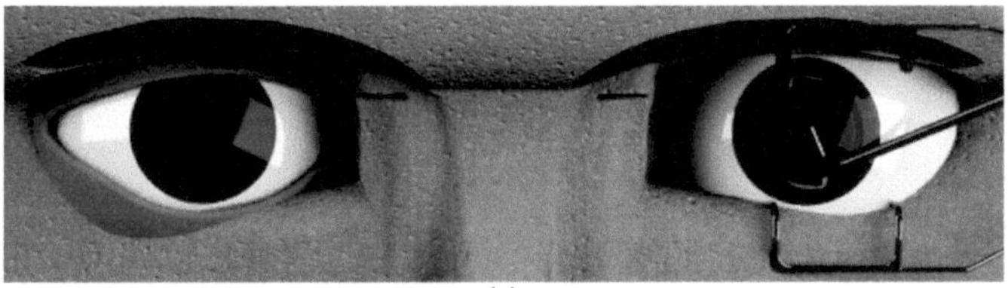

(c)

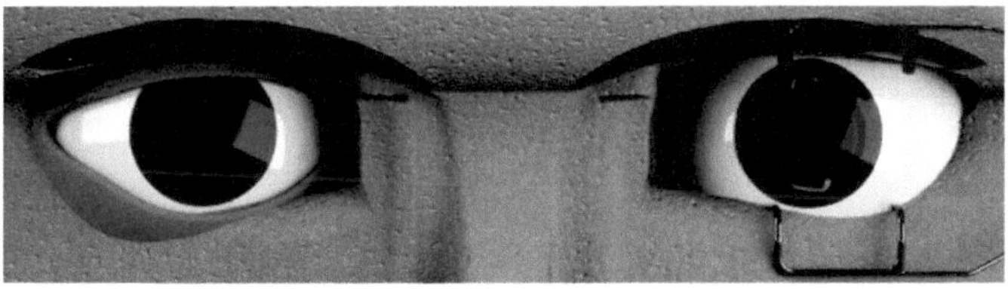

(d)

**Figure 3.42** The proposed robotic system implanting an artificial IOL.

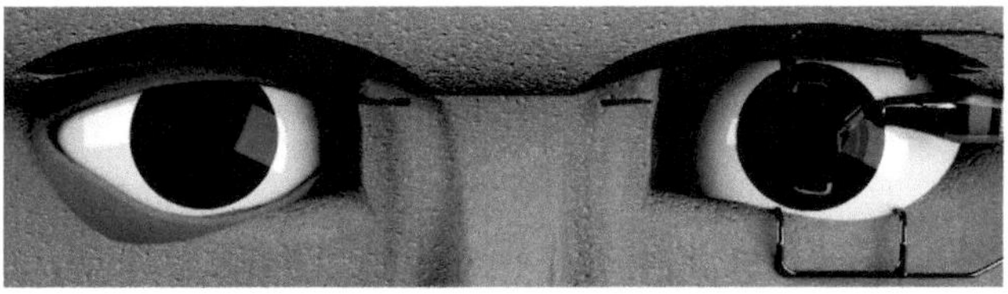

**Figure 3.43** The proposed robotic system removing viscoelastic gel.

9. *Wound sealing/hydration (if needed)*. Thus, the proposed robotic cataract surgery system should be capable of implementing all these steps under supervisory control of the microsurgeon. Additional details are given below: occasionally, a peripheral iridectomy may be performed to minimize the risk of pupillary block glaucoma (Fig. 3.44). An opening through the iris can be fashioned manually (surgical iridectomy) or with a laser (called yttrium aluminum garnet [YAG] laser iridotomy). Laser peripheral iridotomy may be performed either prior to or following cataract surgery. The eye will have mostly recovered within a week, and complete recovery should be expected in about a month. The patient should not participate in contact/extreme sports until cleared to do so by the eye surgeon.

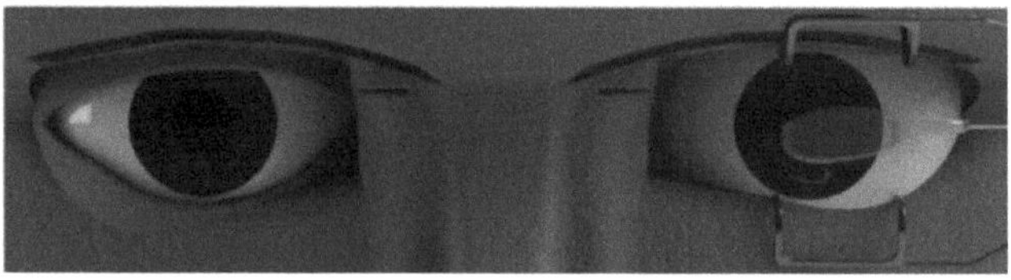

**Figure 3.44** Iridectomy with the proposed robotic system.

In conclusion, all steps involved in cataract removal are feasible with the proposed robotic system. With its 18 degrees of freedom and high precision, this master–slave robot is ideal for any type of high-precision intraocular surgery.

## Problem Set

1. Describe "ophthalmic surgery" and why robots are helpful in performing these operations?
2. Name some ophthalmic surgeries.
3. Describe glaucoma, refractive and vitreoretinal surgeries.
4. Describe the proposed robotic system for use in ophthalmology. Explain all major parts' functions.
5. What is the logic behind proposing a system with this configuration for use in intraocular surgeries?

6. What are the degrees of freedom of the proposed surgical system?
7. What features are incorporated in the proposed system?
8. What are cataracts?
9. How are cataracts treated?
10. What are the steps of phacoemulsification? Describe them.
11. Generate the 3D workspace of the developed surgical system using the derived equations in Chapter 3.
12. Generate the motion trajectory of the tip of the surgical instrument using the equations derived in Chapter 3 with a number of arbitrary set of constraints.

## Chapter 4

# Deployable Laparoscopic Robotic Surgical System

## 4.1 Introduction to Laparoscopic and Robotic Laparoscopic Surgery

Minimally invasive surgical techniques have emerged as a trend in medicine with more advantages over conventional methods, such as short recovery time for the patient, reduced pain due to smaller incisions, and less hemorrhaging. Laparoscopy is an endoscopic surgical operation in the abdomen or pelvis through small incisions with the use of a camera (Fig. 4.1[1]). Typically, a number of small openings (three to six) with a size of 0.5–1.5 cm are made on the body of a patient through which surgical instruments are inserted. These instruments include a laparoscope, which is a long, thin instrument with a light source at the tip of it to illuminate the inside of the abdomen or pelvis. The laparoscope is also equipped with a lens at its tip that takes images and sends them to a video monitor through optical fibers for the surgeon and other staff to view in real time. The abdomen is filled with carbon dioxide ($CO_2$) through a special needle, which is inserted just below the navel. This gas is very helpful in separating the organs inside the abdominal cavity and making it easier for the surgeon to see the organs during

[1]http://www.cincinnatifertility.com/infertility-treatment/laparoscopy

*Robotic Surgery: Smart Materials, Robotic Structures, and Artificial Muscles*
Mohsen Shahinpoor and Siavash Gheshmi

ISBN 978-981-4316-23-1 (Hardcover), 978-981-4463-51-5 (eBook)
www.panstanford.com

laparoscopy. The gas is removed at the end of the procedure. Figure 4.2 compares conventional and laparoscopic cholecystectomy.

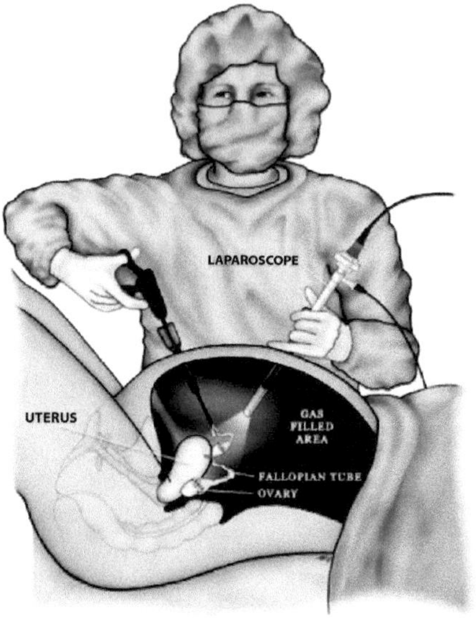


**Figure 4.1** Laparoscopic surgical procedure.

Robot-assisted surgery has introduced a new era of minimally invasive surgical procedures and is going to revolutionize the entire field of conventional open surgery by introducing methods that are far less invasive and by offering many fundamental clinical improvements that are outstanding for both patients and surgeons. Robots are also being used more to help with laparoscopic surgeries. Significant research has been conducted on the utilization of robots in surgical procedures, the outcome of which has been verified by testing commercial and noncommercial robotic surgical systems. Horgan and Vanuno (2001) published a technical report on the use of robotic systems in laparoscopy in which they concluded that robot-assisted operations are safer and more effective as compared to conventional laparoscopic procedures. Russell H. Taylor and Dan Stoianovici (2003) provide a comprehensive review of robotic surgical systems developed. Sabharwal, Pradhan, and Kumar (2006) evaluated the da Vinci® surgical robot for use in urology, more specifically radical prostatectomy, renal surgery, and adrenalectomy. Their study shows that the da Vinci® system could successfully be utilized in urological surgeries and has led to a set of standards for robot-assisted operations. Indeed, the use of the da Vinci® robot in a number of other surgeries, such as general surgery and cardiac surgery, has been successful as well (Hemal and Menon, 2004). Recent technological advents in video imaging, endoscopic techniques, and instrumentation have converted a number of manual operations into robotic ones.

Robotic telescopic assistance with systems such as AESOP® or robotic procedural laparoscopy with systems such as da Vinci® or ZEUS® are two frequent approaches to perform minimally invasive surgeries (Shew, Ostlie, and Holcomb, 2003). The former is a rather semiautomated method due to manual adjustments of optical fiber endoscopic cameras. The latter, on the other hand, involves the use of teleoperative methods, where the robotic system is of a master–slave type and the surgeon performs surgery from a distance. These systems have been widely used in cardiology, gynecology (Yildrim, 2010), urology (Ashish Sabharwal, Pradhan, and Kumar, 2006; Casale and Kojima, 2009), general surgery, laparoscopy, etc.

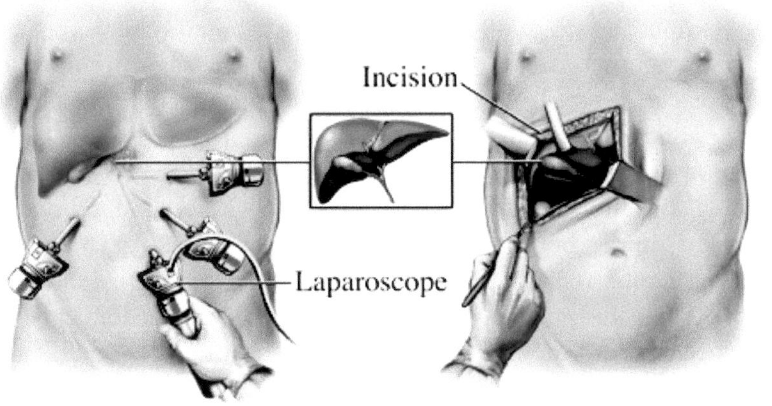


**Figure 4.2** Laparoscopic and conventional cholecystectomy.[2]

A teleoperative robotic system comprises two fundamental units. One is an ergonomically designed surgical master station housing the surgeon as the master of surgical robotic operation. He/she sits on a chair and uses a pair of multi-degree-of-freedom controllers

[2]http://etsyitemoftheday.com/gallbladders/

for manipulation of a number of distant robotic end effectors and an endoscopic camera. The video monitor enables the surgeon to observe and control the surgical operation on the body of the patient. The other major unit is a robotic slave system that actually performs the surgery on the patient's body by delivering different surgical end effectors into his or her body to do surgical tasks such as gripping, cutting, and suturing. The end effectors are equipped with different sensors to receive continuous information on force and displacements.

Many patents and patent applications have been reported in connection with robotic surgery. Van Der Brug, Bliek, and Gerritsen (1999) developed an image-guided surgical system to show a surgeon the position of a surgical instrument in an operating area in the body of a patient during a surgical procedure. Diolaiti (2010) describes a control system for a minimally invasive surgical system that could be used as both a centralized and a distributed system. As a centralized system, a motion controller receives master inputs, sensor inputs from the slave arms, and optimization inputs and uses them to send out control signals to an instrument, an imaging system, and a guide tube controller. As a distributed system, a control and transform processor receives data from a master arm controller, an instrument controller, an imaging system controller, and a guide tube controller and distributes data received from one controller to the other controllers. The other controllers use the received data, along with the optimization goals, to control associated slave arms in a distributed but coordinated way. Nowlin et al. (2011) introduce surgical robotic devices, systems, and methods that use surgical robotic linkages that may have more degrees of freedom than an associated surgical end effector in space. Pivoting of a tool about an aperture site is achieved through a software-based tool motion control. Linkages can take multiple configurations to deliver the end effector to a given position, which helps with collision prevention. Larkin and Shafer (2011) introduce a surgical instrument, which includes articulated arms having a distal end, a proximal end, and one joint region disposed between the distal and proximal ends; an optical fiber bend sensor and a detection system coupled to it; and a control system comprising a servo controller for effectuating movement of the arm. The compact, flexible, snake-like structure of the instrument gives additional dexterity to the manipulator.

## 4.2 AESOP®, ZEUS®, and da Vinci®: First Methods and Systems in Robotic Laparoscopy

### 4.2.1 AESOP®

AESOP® (Fig. 4.3) was developed by Computer Motion, Goleta, CA. With a Food and Drug Administration (FDA) clearance in 1994, it became the first robot to assist in a surgery. AESOP® was released in several generations, such as 1000, 2000, and 3000, with the latest models having more features, such as a voice recognition system to receive voice commands from a surgeon. Hermes®, a platform designed with the purpose of networking the operating room (OR) through voice controls, enables a surgeon to fully and directly control the surgical equipment (Horgan and Vanuno, 2001). A normal surgical procedure with AESOP® would include making three to five small incisions in a patient's body through which an endoscopic camera and robotic instruments are inserted.

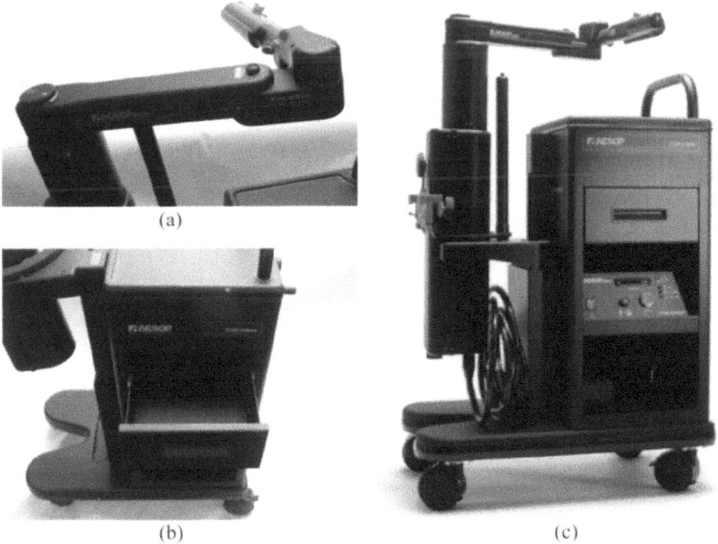

**Figure 4.3** AESOP® 3000 robotic surgical system; different views.

### 4.2.2 Zeus®

Zeus® (Fig. 4.4) is a robotic system developed by the same company, Computer Motion. It includes three interactive arms: the first arm is voice activated and controls the laparoscope; the other two arms are controlled via joysticks at the surgeon's workstation and manipulate surgical instruments (Horgan and Vanuno, 2001).

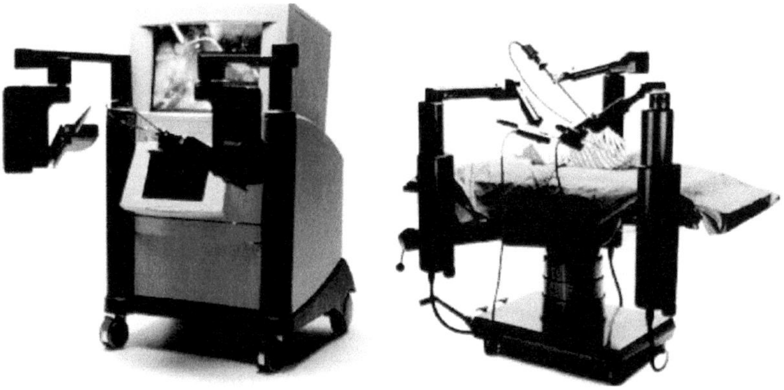

**Figure 4.4** Zeus® robotic surgical system.

### 4.2.3 Da Vinci®

Da Vinci® (Fig. 4.5) is a robotic system developed by Intuitive Surgical, Sunnydale, CA. It consists of two main entities, a surgeon's console housing the surgeon as the master of the surgical operation and a slave robot composed of four robotic arms. The robot is under full control of the surgeon and is never autonomous. The surgeon is provided with a stereoscopic and panoramic view of the surgical scene and controls the movements of the robotic arms via joysticks in the surgeon's console. In the slave robot, which actually performs the surgery on the patient's body, one of the arms positions an endoscopic camera with two lenses inside the body, while the other three manipulate surgical instruments and act as a gripper, a scalpel, scissors, a bovie, and unipolar or bipolar electrocautery instruments. The da Vinci® system also includes multiple, redundant safety features to reduce human error possibilities.

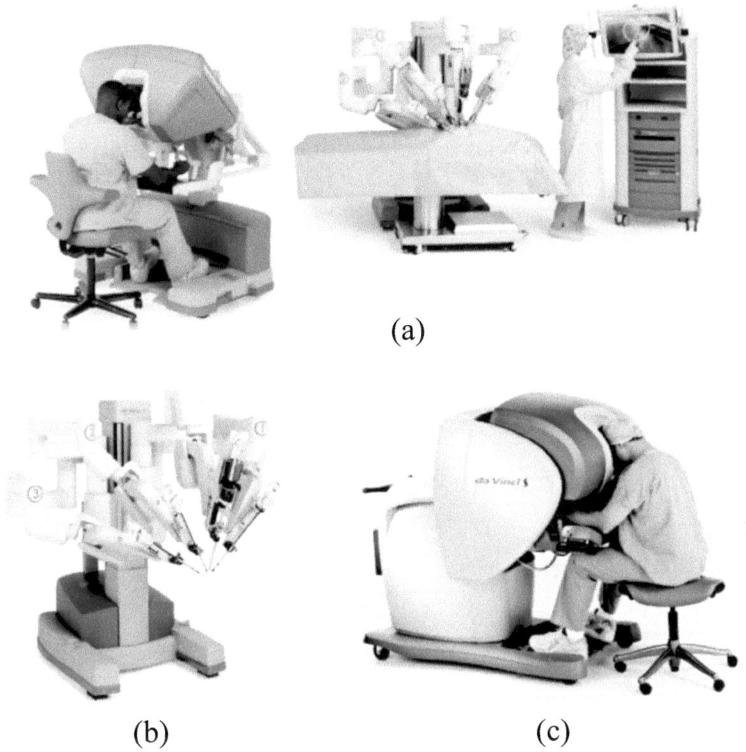


**Figure 4.5** Da Vinci® robotic surgical system. (a) The whole system, (b) the surgical arm cart, and (c) the surgeon's console.

In conventional laparoscopy, the surgeon operates while standing, using handheld, long-shafted instruments, and to see an image of the target anatomy, he/she has to look up and away from the instruments to a close-by 2D monitor. The surgeon also depends on his/her assistant to position the camera correctly. In contrast, the da Vinci® system is developed to enhance conventional laparoscopy. Using the ergonomically designed da Vinci® system, a physician can operate from a seated position at the surgeon's console, with eyes and hands positioned in line with the instruments. The surgeon's hand movements, to manipulate the instruments or to reposition the camera, are scaled, filtered, and translated into more precise micromovements of the instruments, which operate through small incisions in the body. Figure 4.6 illustrates a typical scene of a surgical procedure with the help of the da Vinci® robotic system. In the following section, we will describe different sections and parts of a robotic surgical system with the help of da Vinci® as the only widely used commercial robotic system for use in surgeries.

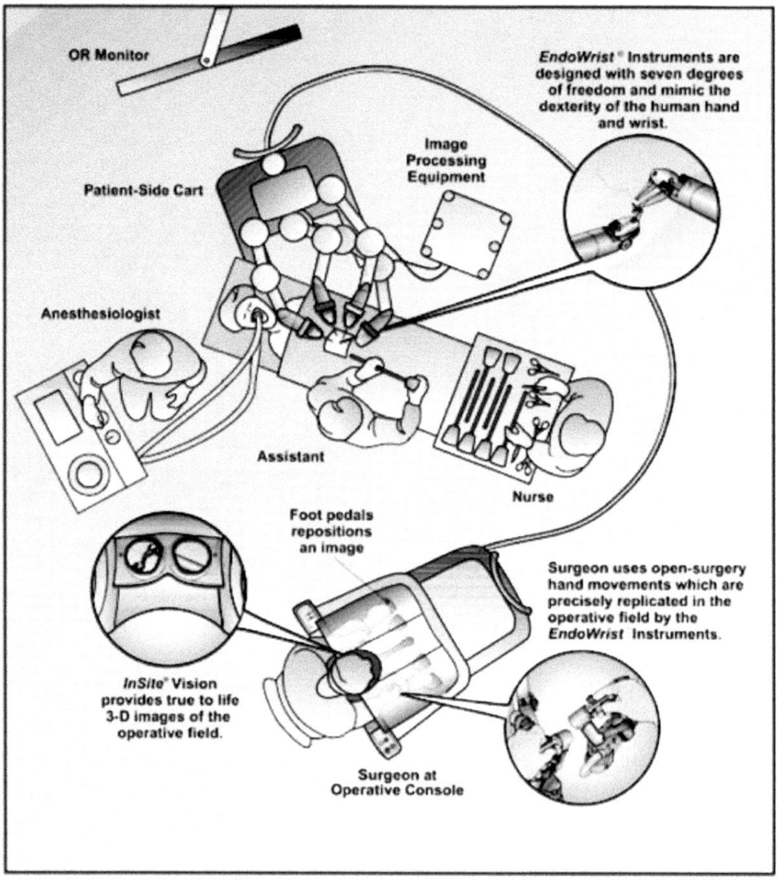


**Figure 4.6** The da Vinci® robotic surgical system in an OR.

Any robot-assisted surgical system should comprise five main units: a surgeon console, image-processing equipment, surgical instruments, a slave robot, and an endoscopic camera (Fig. 4.7). In the following section, we will elaborate on each of these units, exploiting the da Vinci® robotic surgical system–associated items, which are:

- Surgeon console
- Image-processing equipment
- EndoWrist® instruments
- Surgical arm cart
- High-resolution 3D endoscope

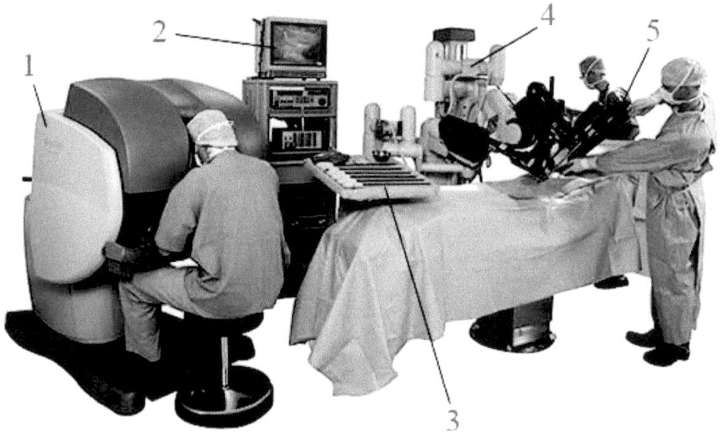


**Figure 4.7** The da Vinci® robotic surgical system main units. (1) A surgeon console, (2) image-processing equipment, (3) EndoWrist® instruments, (4) a surgical arm cart, and (5) a high-resolution 3D endoscope.

### 4.2.3.1 Surgeon console

The surgeon sits comfortably at the da Vinci® console (Fig. 4.8) and looks at a generated panoramic image of the surgical operation through two eyeholes. To operate, the surgeon uses the two foot pedals and two hand controllers to manipulate the slave robot arms. As the surgeon moves the controllers, the slave robot responds accordingly in real time, scaling, filtering, and translating his/her hand, wrist, and finger movements into micromovements of surgical instruments at the patient-side cart.

The master controls are located below the display, and the hand and eye are aligned naturally for optimal performance. The foot switch panel gives the surgeon the flexibility to perform a multitude of tasks such as exchanging different types of surgical instruments. The surgeon is provided with an immersive stereo viewer for more precision.

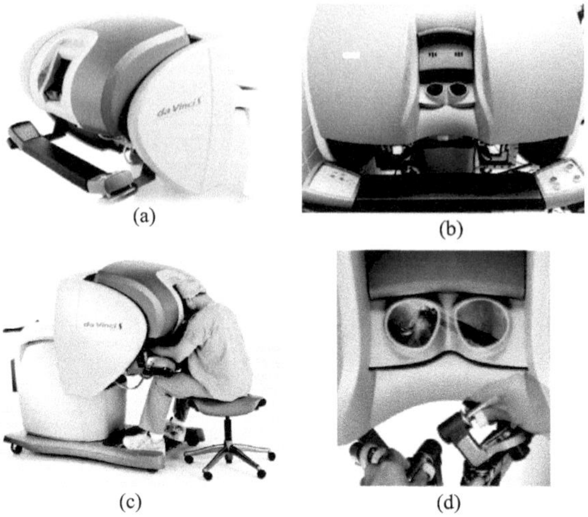


**Figure 4.8** The da Vinci® surgeon console; different views.

An integrated surgeon touchpad is used to perform comprehensive control of video, audio, and system settings. Moreover, audio/visual feedback constantly notifies the surgeon and the OR team of system status and functions (Fig. 4.9).

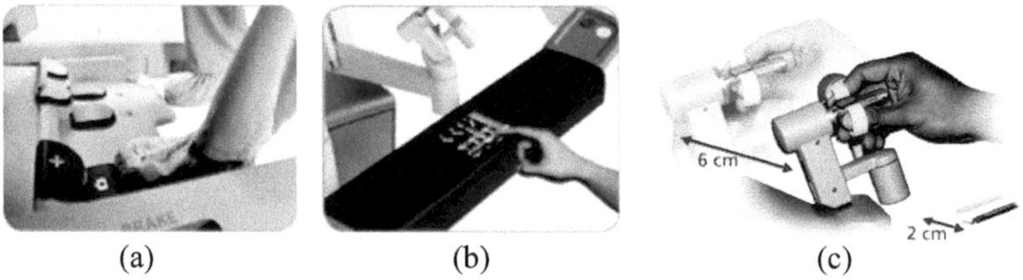


**Figure 4.9** The da Vinci® surgeon console; different sections. (a) A surgeon touchpad, (b) a fingertip controller and scaling feature, and (c) foot pedals.

*Dual console capability* (Fig. 4.10) offers training and collaboration during a minimally invasive surgical intervention. In collaboration mode, each surgeon sits at his/her own console and views the same image of the operation. Two surgeons of the same or different specialties can collaborate on a single case, exchanging control of the instrument arms and the endoscope at any time. In training mode, the teaching surgeon can give control of the instruments to the resident/fellow at appropriate times. This see-and-repeat model of instruction catalyzes the learning procedures.

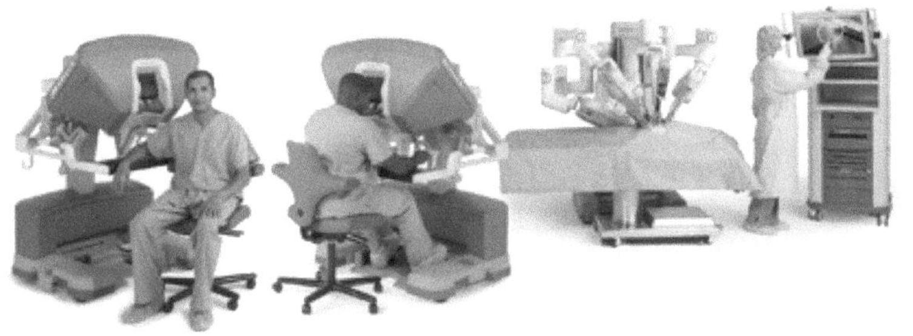

**Figure 4.10** The da Vinci® surgeon dual console.

#### 4.2.2.2 Image-processing equipment

The slave robot on a patient's side inserts a high-definition (HD) 3D endoscope into the body of the patient to capture images of his/her anatomy and send them to image-processing equipment, which provides a true-to-life image of the patient's anatomy. A large view of the operating field with natural depth perception is shown on a monitor available on the vision cart. A magnification feature allows surgeons to handle surgeries more easily and efficiently, especially in operations with limited space, such as the chest and abdomen (Figs. 4.11 and 4.12).

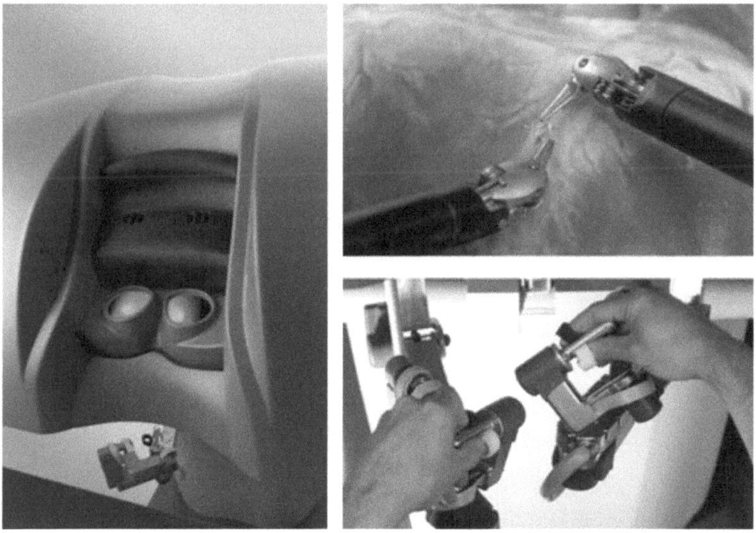

**Figure 4.11** The da Vinci® surgeon console vision system.

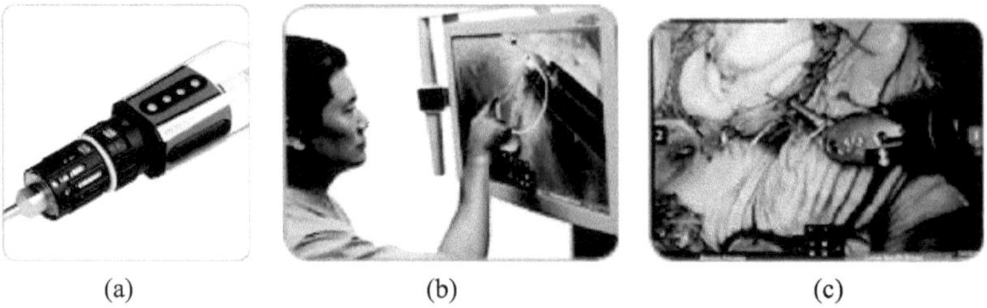


**Figure 4.12** The da Vinci® image-processing equipment. (a) A wide-screen touch screen, (b) visual resolution (1080i HD), (c) a 3D HD camera head.

#### 4.2.3.3 EndoWrist® instruments

Da Vinci® EndoWrist® surgical instruments are the ones in contact with target organs and perform different surgical tasks. These instruments include needle drivers, graspers, scalpels, scissors, monopolar and bipolar cautery instruments, ultrasonic energy instruments, clip appliers, etc. Cannulas (Fig. 4.13) guide surgical instruments into the body to the target organ. They provide easy insertion of surgical instruments into the body without damaging the surrounding tissue and organs due to frequent instrument exchange. A complete list of EndoWrist® surgical instruments, cannulas, etc., is available in *EndoWrist Instrument & Accessory Catalog* released by Intuitive Surgical.

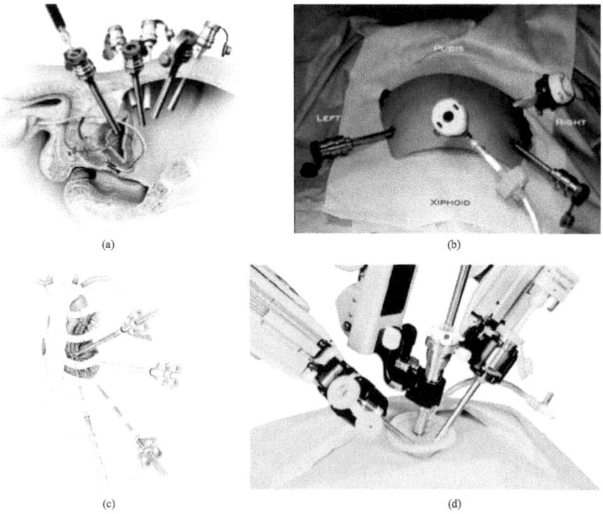


**Figure 4.13** Da Vinci® cannulas; different representations.

EndoWrist® surgical instruments (Figs. 4.14 and 4.15) have 7 degrees of freedom with 90 degrees of articulation, which are inserted into the body through 1–2 cm incisions. These instruments provide the surgeon with more dexterity and precision, which make the operation easier with greater outcomes. The surgeon's hand movements are scaled and transferred to these instruments. They come in two different general sizes, 5 mm and 8 mm.

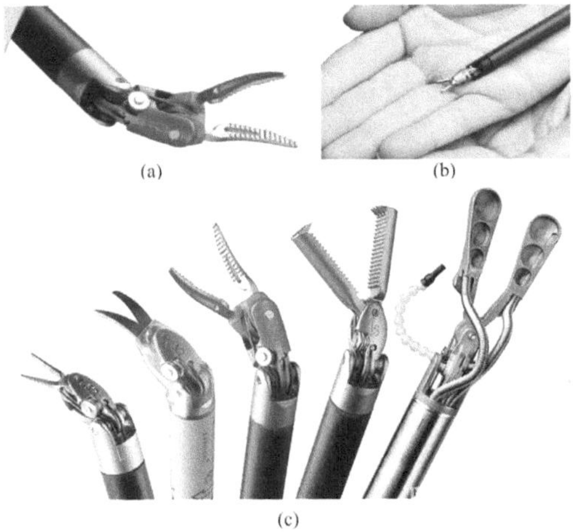


**Figure 4.14** Da Vinci® EndoWrist® surgical instruments; different representations.

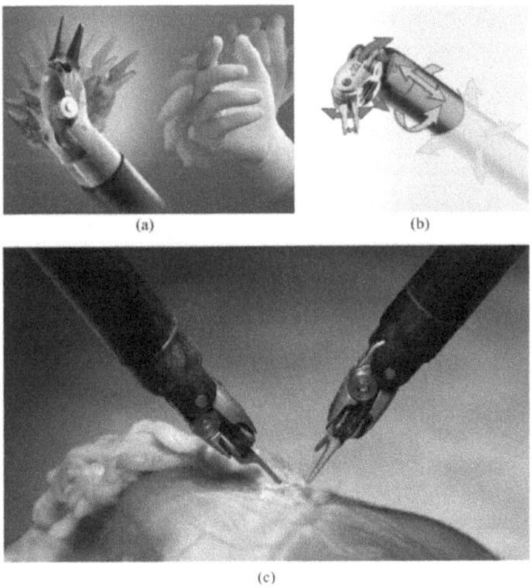


**Figure 4.15** Da Vinci® EndoWrist® surgical instruments. (a) Degrees of freedom, (b) dexterity, and (c) instruments in use.

#### 4.2.3.4 Surgical arm cart

The da Vinci® slave robot has four multiquadrant access arms, three of which hold EndoWrist® surgical instruments (Fig. 4.16). The other arm positions the endoscopic camera. These arms deliver the surgical instruments into the patient's body under full control of the surgeon and move around a fixed pivot point to reduce trauma to the patient.

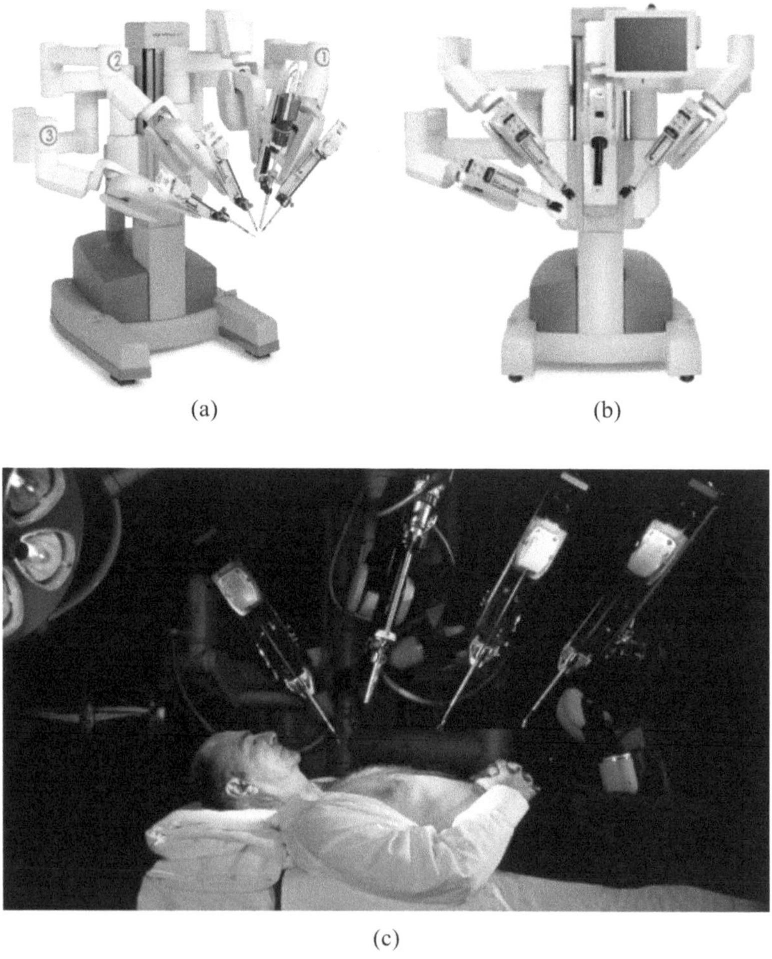


**Figure 4.16** The da Vinci® surgical arm cart.

### 4.2.3.5 High-resolution 3D endoscope

The endoscopic camera that is inserted into the patient's body to capture image of the surgery is shown in Fig. 4.17. There are two types of endoscopes released by Intuitive Surgical, 0° and 30° stereo endoscopes.

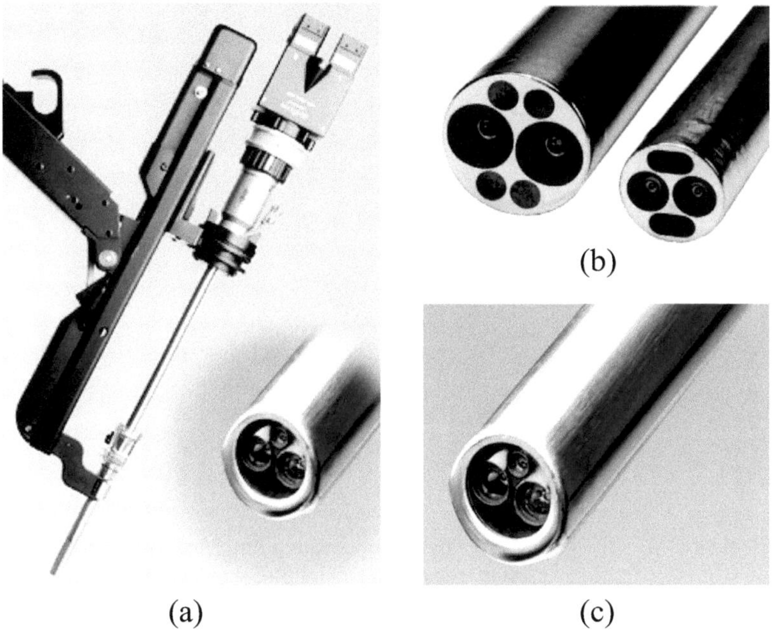


**Figure 4.17** Da Vinci® high-resolution 3D endoscopes.

Figure 4.18 is a pictorial presentation of the benefits of robot-assisted minimally invasive surgeries to conventional ones and is as follows: (a) multi-incision laparoscopy versus single-site da Vinci® surgery, (b) open hysterectomy incision versus da Vinci® hysterectomy incision, (c) da Vinci® thyroidectomy versus open thyroidectomy, (d) open kidney surgery incision versus da Vinci® surgery incision, (e) open surgical incision versus da Vinci® mitral valve repair incision, and (f) open prostatectomy incision versus da Vinci® prostatectomy incision.

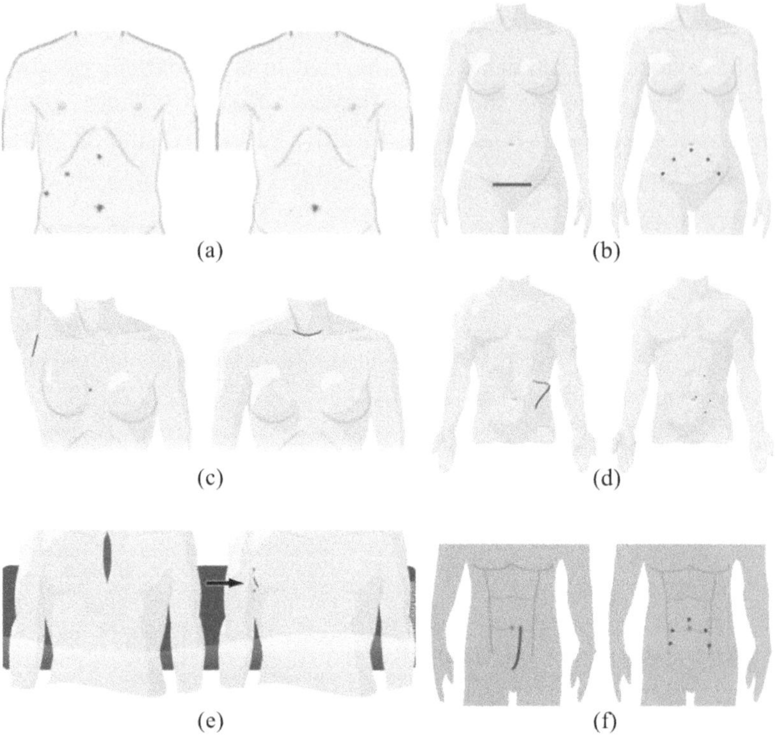


**Figure 4.18** Difference between conventional surgical procedures and robot-assisted ones with the help of the da Vinci® robot.

The following picture (Fig. 4.19) shows the outcome of a robot-assisted surgery with the help of the da Vinci® Surgical System.

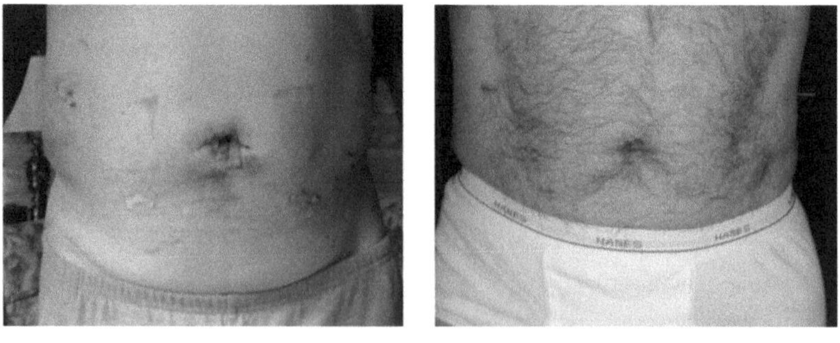

**Figure 4.19** Result of a robot-assisted surgery with the help of the da Vinci® robot.

Robotic surgical systems are still under continuous improvements. One major issue yet to be solved is the big size of the surgeon's console and surgical slave robot. The da Vinci® Surgical System occupies a considerable amount of working space in the OR and makes it inconvenient for surgeons and nurses to be around the surgical bed, when necessary. It also takes up a lot of useful space in the OR when not working. Thus, the introduction of a new system that takes less space of the OR in both working and nonworking modes is essential. We developed a new type of robotic surgical system at the University of Maine, which is currently under provisional patent status (#61718822). Our focus is on the introduction of compact alternatives for sections 1 and 4 of the da Vinci® system, which are the surgeon's console and the surgical arm cart, respectively.

In the following section, we give an introduction to deployable structures as the base of our proposed robotic surgical system.

## 4.3 Deployable Structures

### 4.3.1 Introduction to Deployable Structures

Deployable structures that can adjust their configuration to a predetermined size or shape under specific operating conditions have found a great deal of interest in various fields of industry (Gantes and Konitopoulou, 2004). The term "smart deployable structure" refers to the capability of such structures to switch from one configuration to another to meet any engineering requirements. Most deployable structures that have been developed are open-closed structures that fulfill their functionality after full deployment. They are specifically used for efficient packing during storage and transportation. Well-known examples of these bi-state structures range from small structures, such as deployable tents, to large civil structures, such as retractable roofs of sports stadiums (Pellegrino and Calladine, 1986), (Kassabian, You, and Pellegrino, 1999). Highly engineered examples include space structures such as solar arrays and antennas on spacecraft in which compactness, light weight, and easy deployment are necessary for such structures to be compactly stowed for launch and then autonomously deployed to their final configuration. Currently, the final deployed shape of such structures is limited to simple linear or circular geometry. However, development of structures that are capable of deploying to different desired curves may have a large number of applications ranging from biomedical applications such as gastrointestinal robotic surgery to complex curvilinear deployable space structures.

Several mechanisms have been proposed to obtain shape-morphing structures (Del Grosso and Basso, 2010). One example is truss structures in which some of the truss links are replaced with linear displacement actuators and can be deployed from a tightly packed form to the functional state (Onoda, Fu, and Minesugi, 1996; Sofla, Elzey, and Wadley, 2009). Another example is tensegrity mechanisms, which are lightweight space structures consisting of compression members surrounded by a network of tension members (Fest et al., 2003). These mechanisms change their shape on the basis of the static or dynamic equilibrium state.

Scissor-like element (SLE) structures are an important class of smart structures that are unique in terms of simplicity, deploying mechanism, and application (Fig. 4.20).

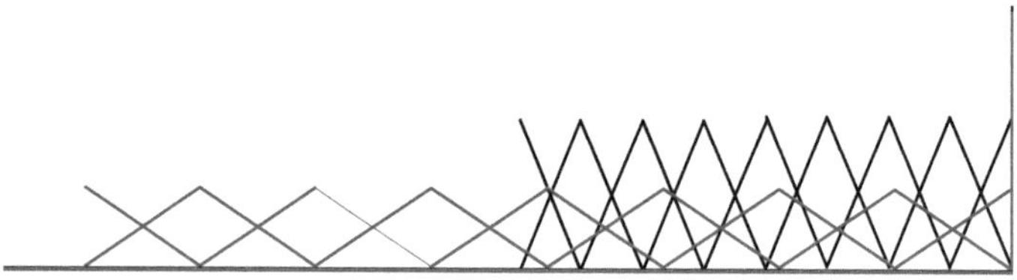

**Figure 4.20** Linear deployment of the SLE mechanism.

SLE structures are mechanical configurations consisting of a set of rigid elements connected to each other at an intermediate point by revolute joints. Normally, SLE structures are one-degree-of-freedom mechanisms that deploy to the final shape with high accuracy using an actuator that controls the entire shape. Ease of transportation, light weight, space-saving quality, high strength, and stability against external loadings are important advantages of these smart structures that have made their application promising in grabbers, robotic end effectors, structural roofs, and space structures. An outstanding application of SLE-based mechanisms has been introduced by Pinero (1961), who developed a full-size foldable theater, which arrived at the site on a single wheelbarrow and was then unfolded on the basis of an SLE mechanism. Hoberman (1990, 1991, 2007) made considerable advance in the design of retractable structures based on SLE mechanisms when he discovered the simple angulated element.

Interestingly, SLE structures can also be found in biological structures at the cellular level. For instance, the DNA structure exhibits self-assembling into an expanded pattern, which is similar to that of an SLE (Fig. 4.21) (Strong, 2004).

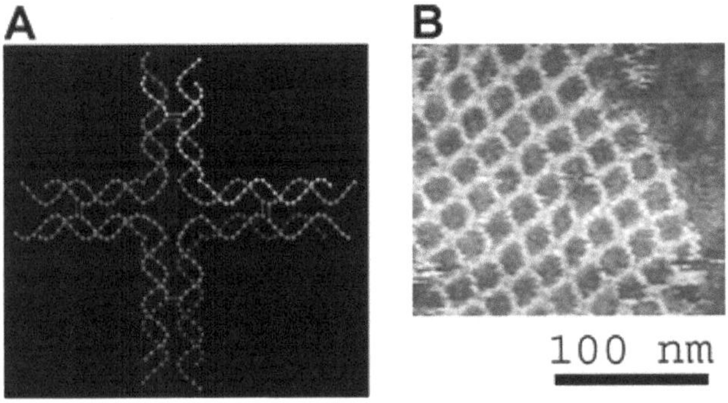


**Figure 4.21** The DNA structure one the left (schematically shown) will self-assemble into the structure visualized by atomic force microscopy on the right (Strong, 2004).

Chen et al. (2002) suggested a new design based on diagonals (web struts) and lower chords to enhance the structural stiffness of deployable structures. Tsutomu and Tokai (1997) presented a cable scissors arch (CSA) based on a scissor mechanism in which three-hinged arch scissors and flexible cables were used to control the shape. Shahinpoor (1996) introduced a novel design of multifingered robotic grabbers capable of rapidly deploying their robotic fingers for grabbing tasks. An interesting case is presented in a paper submitted by Maden, Korkmaza, and Akgünb (2011) in which the authors discuss basic typologies, geometric principles, design rules, and constraints of planar scissor structural mechanisms (SSMs). In this paper they further develop trigonometric calculation methods for different types of SSMs, using a deductive approach, and relate these concepts to architectural applications, where traditional inductive methods are inappropriate (Maden, Korkmaza, and Akgünb, 2011).

### 4.3.2 Geometrical Characteristics of Circular Deployable Structures

Assuming all the links have the same length, the final deployed shape of an SLE structure depends on the location of its revolute joints. If all of the links are pivoted to each other at the center of each link (zero off-center) the structure deploys linearly; otherwise the shape of the structure will turn into a curvilinear pattern. In case of a constant off-center value of all hinge points, the final deployed shape will be circular after deployment. Figures 4.22a and 4.22b show an example of a constant off-center structure before and after deployment, respectively. Basically, one end of the first link set is pivoted to the ground, while the other end is actuated using a linear pneumatic, hydraulic, or electric actuator acting on a straight horizontal line. It can be seen that the trajectory of points on different links does not follow a circular pattern, showing that the radius of curvature of the mechanism varies as it expands. For a circular expansion, all the pivot points are located off-center, which causes the structure to move while following a curve.

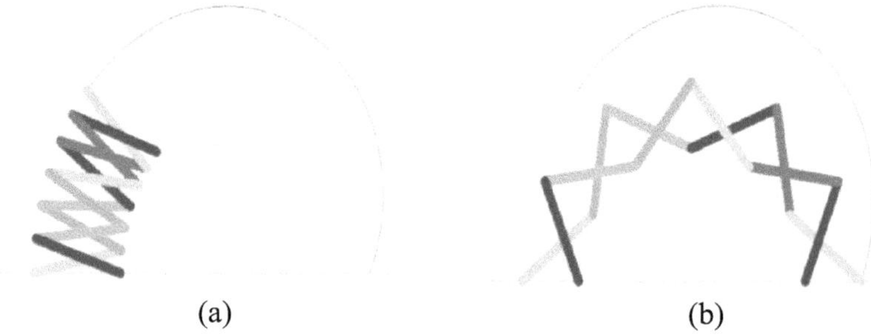

**Figure 4.22** Circular deployable structure (a) in closed mode and (b) in deployed mode.

Referring to Fig. 4.23, the dependency of overall radius on amount of deployment can be calculated by the following equation:

$$R = \frac{a.\sin\theta}{\sin\left[\dfrac{\theta - \sin^{-1}\left(\dfrac{a}{b}.\sin\theta\right)}{2}\right]} \tag{4.1}$$

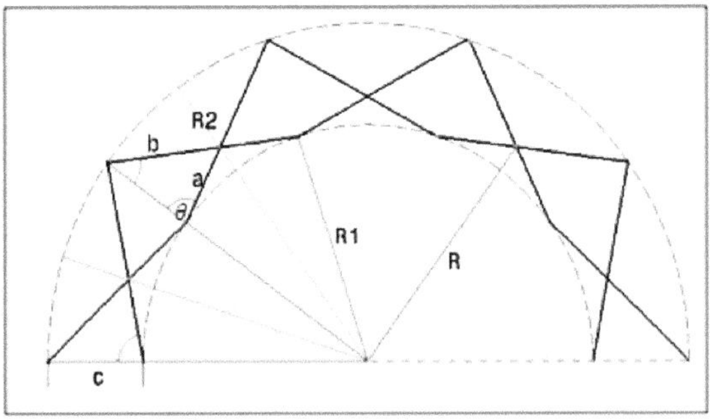


**Figure 4.23** Dependency of the deployed radius on the offset and the amount of deployment.

As it is shown, the final radius of the deployed circle depends on the amount of offset, $a/b$. In the special case of $a = b$, the deployed radius $R$ goes to infinity, which shows the structure deploys linearly.

On the basis of this analysis, it can be concluded that by adjusting the offset value of the pivot points, we can control the final deployed shape of these types of structures. Depicted in the next section is a geometrical method to adjust the location of the pivot points in order for the mechanism to be deployed to a predesigned shape.

It should be mentioned that a range of dexterous grabbers can be designed on the basis of these deployable mechanisms. An important application of this concept can be found in the field of robotics where improving the dexterity of end effectors during the grabbing is of high importance. In Figs. 4.24 and 4.25 the 3D models of designed multifingered grabbers in the role of robotic grabbers are demonstrated.

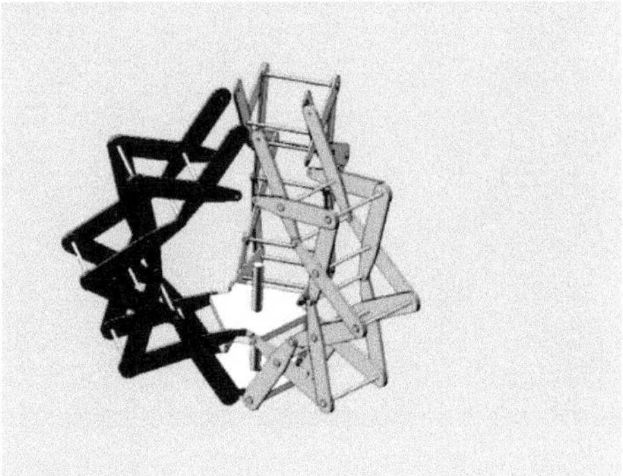

**Figure 4.24** Three-finger robotic grabber based on an SLE in deployed mode.

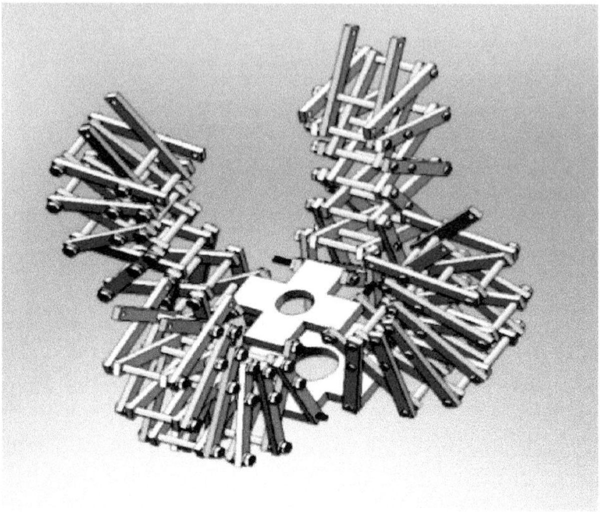

**Figure 4.25** Four-finger robotic grabber based on an SLE in deployed mode.

An important advantage of these types of deployable grabbers over other types of grabbers is that these mechanisms can be deployed using only one actuator. Two experimental models were fabricated on the basis of these designs, and successful deployment is demonstrated in Figs. 4.26 and 4.27.

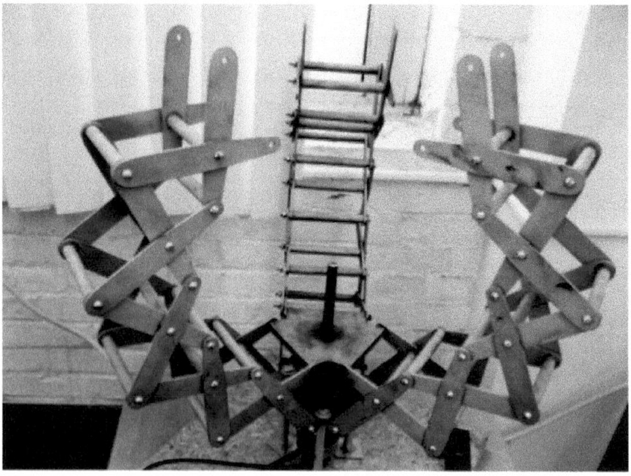

**Figure 4.26** An experimental model for a three-finger robotic grabber based on an SLE in deployed mode.

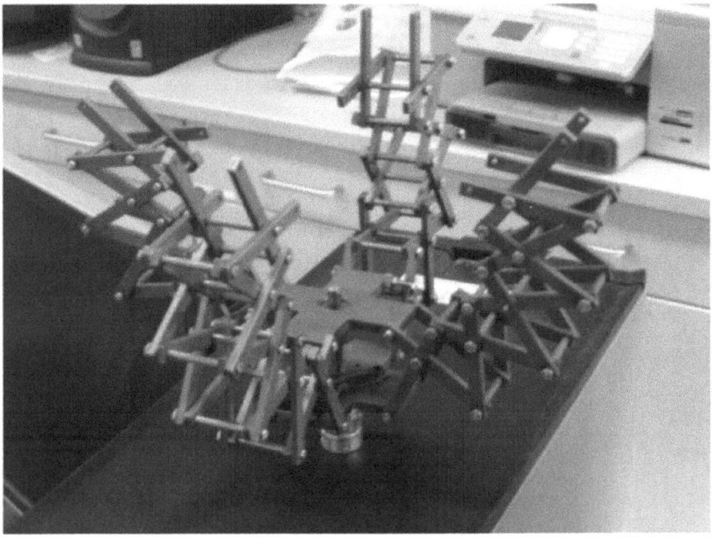

Figure 4.27 An experimental model for a four-finger robotic grabber based on an SLE in deployed mode.

### 4.3.3 Geometrical Characteristics of Curvilinear Deployable Structures

In Fig. 4.28, a design process to achieve a desired final deployed shape is shown. Two circular curves are attached to each other, and an offset of each curve is created. By equally partitioning each of the curves and constructing the links lines, it can be seen that the pivot joints offset from one of the strips varies in the transition point of the two circular curves, which allows the deployed shape to be a combination of the two curves.

Figure 4.29a,b demonstrates a virtual simulation of the proposed mechanism using ADAMS software. 26 rigid links have been pivoted by 35 revolute joints, and a point-curve constraint is applied at the end link where the actuation is applied on the constrained point. Basically, a point-curve constraint allows the link to have rotation but constrains a point of the link to move on a selected straight line. In practice, the amount of contraction depends on the width of links; to have a more contracted shape, thinner links are required. In Fig. 4.29a, the total displacement of end effectors is plotted with respect to the actuation displacement. As can be seen, the maximum reaching point of the end link does not necessarily happen at the states of fully closed, fully deployed, or predesigned configuration.

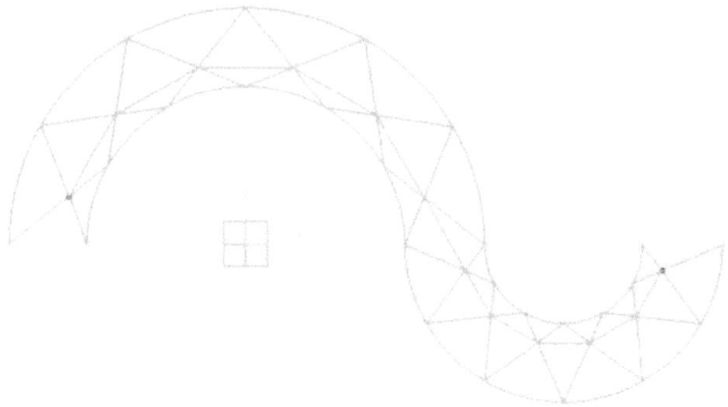

**Figure 4.28** Initial curve, joint location, and path design.

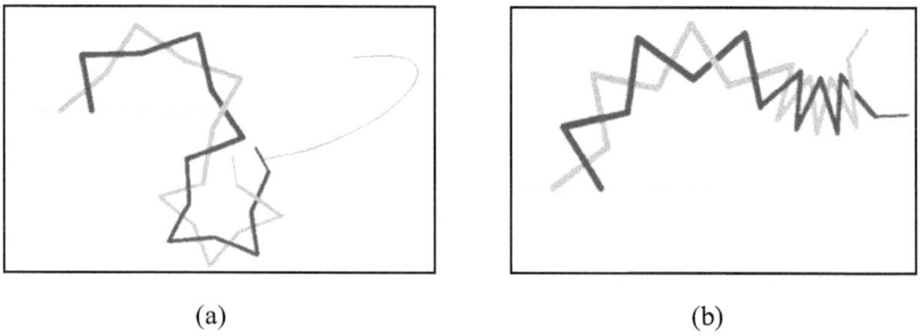

**Figure 4.29** Virtual modeling of the mechanism. (a) Deployed and (b) closed.

Figure 4.30 demonstrates the trajectory of the end effectors with respect to the actuation length variation. Figure 4.31 shows the trajectory of the end effectors during the deployment, which is a complex curvilinear path. As can be observed, during the deployment the radius of curvature at each instant is not constant and depends on the amount of deployment (the angle between two links) for a designed offset value. In the next section, a mathematical model is presented to describe the exact geometry of trajectory and its relation with the actuation length.

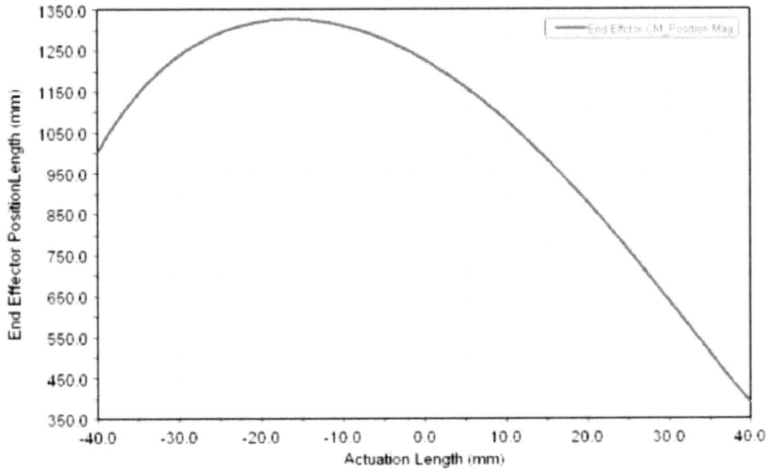


**Figure 4.30** Trajectory of the end effectors vs. the actuation length.

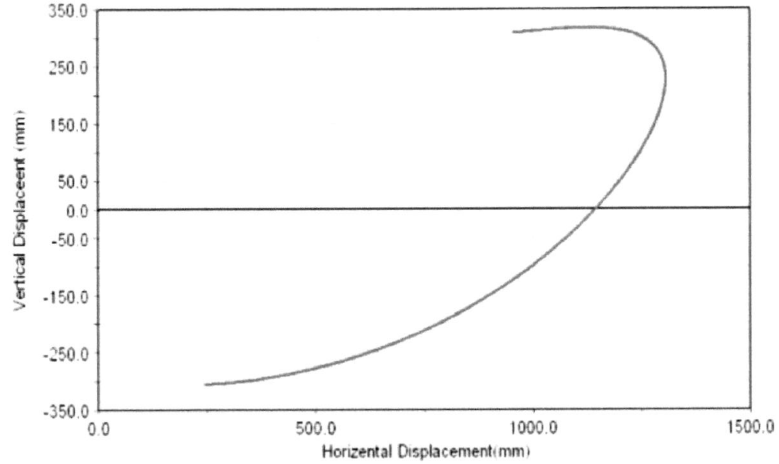


**Figure 4.31** Trajectory of the end effectors during deployment.

Figures 4.32 and 4.33 show the displacement of the last three middle joints in $x$ and $y$ directions, respectively, with respect to time. The actuation length of zero refers to the design configuration of two combined circles, and two other extreme actuation lengths refer to fully closed and fully deployed shapes.

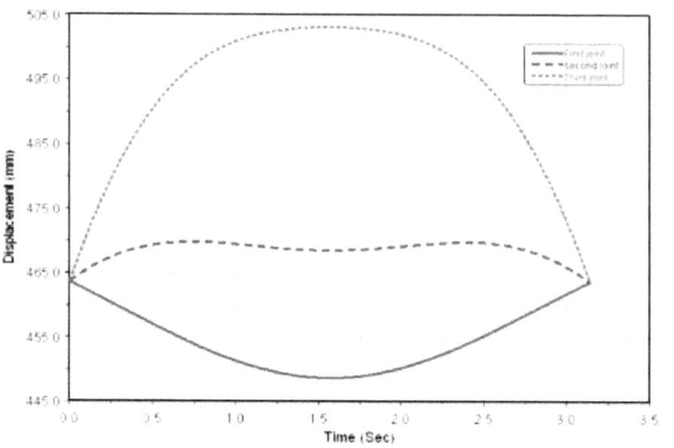


**Figure 4.32** Horizontal displacement of the first three middle joints.

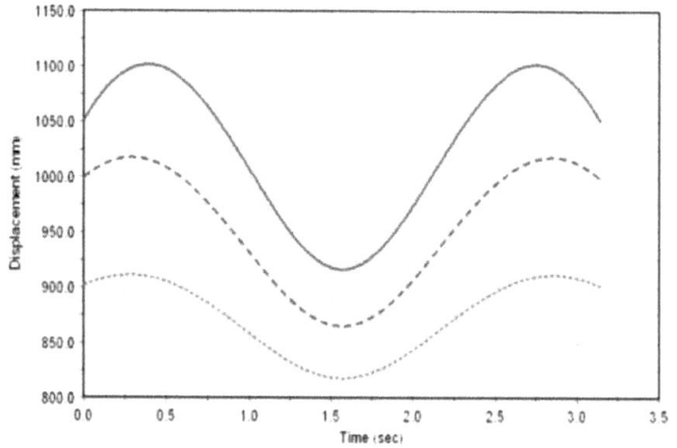


**Figure 4.33** Vertical displacement of the last three middle joints.

## 4.3.4 Mathematical Model of Curvilinear Deployable Structures

This novel curvilinear structure could have many different applications in fields like biomedical engineering and civil engineering. To accomplish a specific task in any of the aforementioned engineering fields, it needs to be guided and deployed into a predetermined curve within a specific period of time. Any curve can be expressed by some mathematical models, and to curvilinearly expand the deployable structure through the curve, some mathematical models for the entire structure are needed so that joints and links are properly actuated to accomplish the specific mission. Geometrical relations between the joints and links of the structure are used to obtain the following mathematical models (Fig. 4.34).

Using simple geometrical relationships between linkages, the position of the $n^{\text{th}}$ pin in the structure can be easily calculated:

$$\begin{bmatrix} X \\ Y \\ 1 \end{bmatrix}_n = \prod_{i=1}^{n} \begin{bmatrix} \cos\theta_{\Delta_i} & -\sin\theta_{\Delta_i} & p_i \\ \sin\theta_{\Delta_i} & \cos\theta_{\Delta_i} & q_i \\ 0 & 0 & 1 \end{bmatrix} \cdot \begin{bmatrix} X_n \\ Y_n \\ 1 \end{bmatrix} \tag{4.2}$$

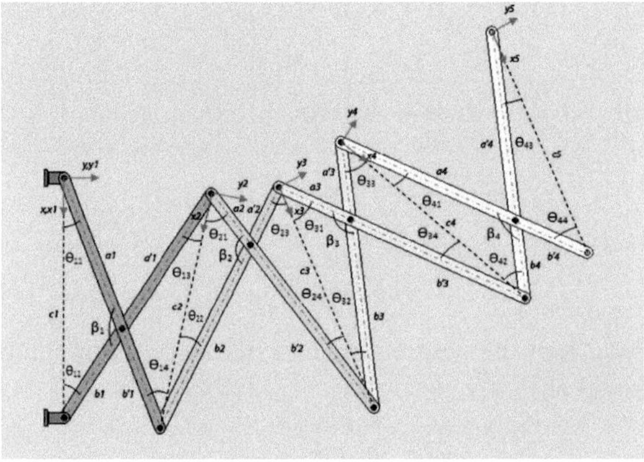

**Figure 4.34** Geometrical properties of a curvilinear deployable structure.

Here all the parameters are illustrated in Fig. 4.34 and are calculated as follows:

$$\cos\theta_{i1} = \left( \frac{a_i^2 + c_i^2 - b_i^2}{2a_i c_i} \right) = \Phi_i^* \tag{4.3}$$

Thus

$$\theta_{i1} = \tan^{-1}\left[ \frac{\sqrt{1-\Phi_i^{*2}}}{\Phi_i^*} \right] \tag{4.4}$$

Similarly, for all angles we have

$$\cos\theta_{i2} = \left( \frac{b_i^2 + c_i^2 - a_i^2}{2b_i c_i} \right) = \Psi_i^* \tag{4.5}$$

$$\theta_{i2} = \tan^{-1}\left[ \frac{\sqrt{1-\Psi_i^{*2}}}{\Psi_i^*} \right] \tag{4.6}$$

$$\beta_i = \pi - \theta_{i1} - \theta_{i2} \tag{4.7}$$

$$\cos\theta_{i3} = \left(\frac{a'^2_i + c_{i+1}{}^2 - b'^2_i}{2a'_i c_{i+1}}\right) = £^*_i \tag{4.8}$$

$$\theta_{i3} = \tan^{-1}\left[\frac{\sqrt{1-£^{*2}_i}}{£^*_i}\right] \tag{4.9}$$

$$\cos\theta_{i3} = \left(\frac{b'^2_i + c_{i+1}{}^2 - a'^2_i}{2b'_i c_{i+1}}\right) = \alpha^*_i \tag{4.10}$$

$$\theta_{i3} = \tan^{-1}\left[\frac{\sqrt{1-\alpha^{*2}_i}}{\alpha^*_i}\right] \tag{4.11}$$

The length of the connecting line of any two opposing joints can be expressed as

$$c_{i+1} = \sqrt{a'^2_i + b'^2_i - 2a'_i b'_i \cos\beta_i} \tag{4.12}$$

The position of the midpin in the $n^{th}$ local coordinate frame is

$$X_n = a_n . \cos\theta_{n1} \tag{4.13}$$

$$Y_n = a_n . \sin\theta_{n1} \tag{4.14}$$

For more simplification, the following substitutions are used in deriving the previously mentioned general equation for the position of the $n^{th}$ pin in the structure:

$$p_{i+1} = c_i - (a'_i + b_i). \cos\theta_{i2} \tag{4.15}$$

$$q_{i+1} = (a'_i + b_i). \sin\theta_{i2} \tag{4.16}$$

$$q_{\Delta_{i+1}} = \theta_{i1} - \theta_{i4} \tag{4.17}$$

$$p_1 = q_1 = \theta_{\Delta_1} = 0 \tag{4.18}$$

The orientation of the dotted line in the $n^{th}$ pair of link is

$$m_{x_n} = \tan\theta_{inc} \tag{4.19}$$

And the orientation of the line perpendicular to the dotted line in the $n^{th}$ pair of link, which is usually the orientation of the end effectors, is

$$m_{y_n} = \frac{-1}{\tan\theta_{\text{inc}}} \tag{4.20}$$

where

$$\theta_{\text{inc}} = \text{Total incline} = \sum_{i=1}^{n-1} \theta_{\Delta_{i+1}} \tag{4.21}$$

The structural characteristics of the mechanism are as follows:

The number of links is 8, and the number of hinge joints is 12. The length of the links is 20 cm. Other parameters are as follows:

Vector of $a_i$ parameters: [153510]

Vector of $a'_i$ parameters: [153510]

Vector of $b_i$ parameters: [5171510]

Vector of $b'_i$ parameters: [5171510]

Using these equations, a kinematic simulation of the deploying process is shown in Figs. 4.35 and 4.36. Figure 4.35 demonstrates the change in the orientation of the end effectors of the last link set, which is the same as the orientation of the line perpendicular to the dotted line of the last link set with respect to the change in the length of linear actuator. Figure 4.36 demonstrates the trajectory of the end joint for a 5.5 cm actuation.

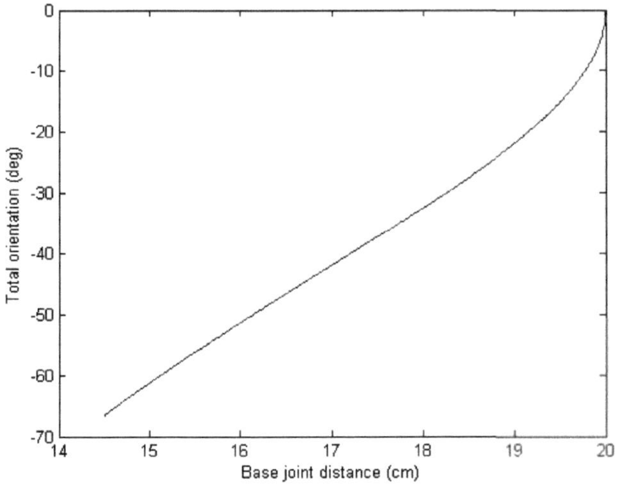


**Figure 4.35** Change in the orientation of the last link vs. change in the displacement of the linear actuator.

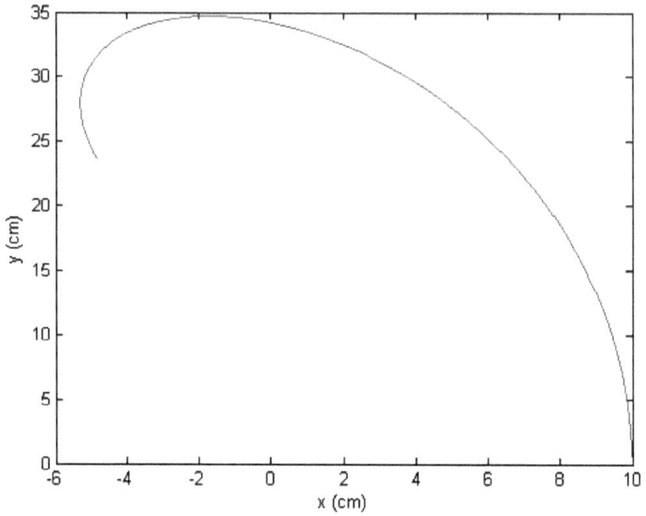


**Figure 4.36** Trajectory of the end joint for a 5.5 cm actuation.

### 4.3.5 Servo-Motorized Intermediate Pins: A Novel Approach

In the previous sections it was shown that by adjusting the offset distance of pivots and lengths of intermediate linkages, the structure can be deployed to any complex shape. This point was proven through a multibody dynamic analysis, and eventually a mathematical model was developed. Similar findings were concluded by Maden, Korkmaza, and Akgünb (2011) in their study, where the authors more specifically discuss the implementation of this method in intricate architectural shapes. Despite the advantages of this model, it lacks flexibility in that pivot points limit the final deployed shape to only one. However, there is a way to overcome this drawback of the simple structure discussed above. This can be achieved through the introduction of a movable pin at the midspan between two ends of each linkage member, said pin being free to move on a screw that connects the two ends of the linkage, while being driven by servo motors installed inside the linkage structure. Two linkage members of a single scissor unit are interconnected at the pins via a connection that permits said movable pins to rotate relative to each other. With the proposed mechanism a highly reconfigurable 2D robot is achieved to cover a sufficient amount of workspace with high dexterity (Fig. 4.37).

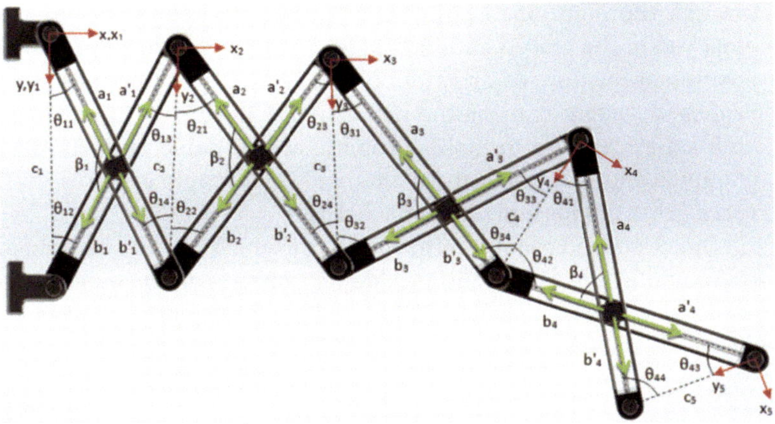

**Figure 4.37** Novel deployable structure with motorized intermediate pins.

## 4.4 Laparoscopic Robotic System with Flexible Deployable Structures

### 4.4.1 Introduction to Our System

In the last section, we proved that an SLE structure with servo-motorized intermediate pins can take any configuration in its deployment plane. As the mathematical models and graphs show, this novel approach toward SLE structures makes it highly dexterous. This highly dexterous 2D robotic system can reach any point in its deploying plane at any orientation through redundant configurations. The system's configuration is obtained through proper control of servo motors to move intermediate pins and open/close the span of the first link set. Different end effectors can be attached on the last link set of this robot. The robot can deliver the end effectors to any point at any orientation.

Mounting this 2D robot on a spherical joint yields a highly dexterous 3D robot capable of reaching any point in 3D space at any orientation. This is achieved through controlling the deployment plane via the spherical joint at the base by tilting and rolling. In 3D space a plane can be defined by a point and a line, the line representing the orientation of the surgical instrument in the space and the point would be the base or the spherical joint by which the deployment plane of the 2D mechanism can be controlled. Therefore, if the deploying plane of the 2D structure coincides with the plane passing through the mentioned point and line, the structure can now be deployed in the aforementioned plane in order to reach the desired position at the desired orientation in 3D space. The core idea of our proposed system is using the novel, highly dexterous 2D structure on a spherical base to make a robotic arm capable of dexterously manipulating surgical instruments and endoscopic cameras in 3D space (Shahinpoor and Gheshmi, 2012).

Our proposed robotic surgical system, which can also be used for training of medical students/residents, consists of two major units, a master surgeon console/station and a robotic surgical slave. We discuss each next.

- *Master surgeon console.* The surgeon's station consists of an ergonomically designed chair, a pair of vision goggles, and a pair of joysticks. The joysticks can be installed on the chair with the help of two platforms. The imaging goggles generate a panoramic view of the surgical scene and assist the surgeon to maintain a natural posture and handle surgeries more easily and comfortably. Imaging features such as magnification further help the surgeon operate more precisely. The surgeon sits on the chair as the master of the robotic surgical procedure and controls the surgical operation via the joysticks. His/her hand movements are scaled, filtered, and translated into movements of surgical instruments snapped onto the robotic slave arms. Using a pair of joysticks and a pair of vision goggles is a space-efficient alternative for current bulky surgeon stations.
- *Robotic surgical slave.* The robotic slave arm is an SLE structure with movable midspan pins mounted on a spherical actuator to change its deployment plane. The relative locations of intermediate pins are altered by servo motors located inside linkages. Figure 4.38 shows a linkage used in the proposed surgical slave robot. As shown in Fig. 4.39, several of these robotic arms can be attached to the sides of the surgical bed in order to manipulate surgical instruments and endoscopic cameras. At the end of the surgery the manipulator arms are contracted and can be placed underneath the surgical bed. Movements of these manipulator arms are under direct control of the surgeon as the master of the surgical intervention. With the proposed robotic surgical slave arms, minimal space is taken up in the surgical room during and after operations.

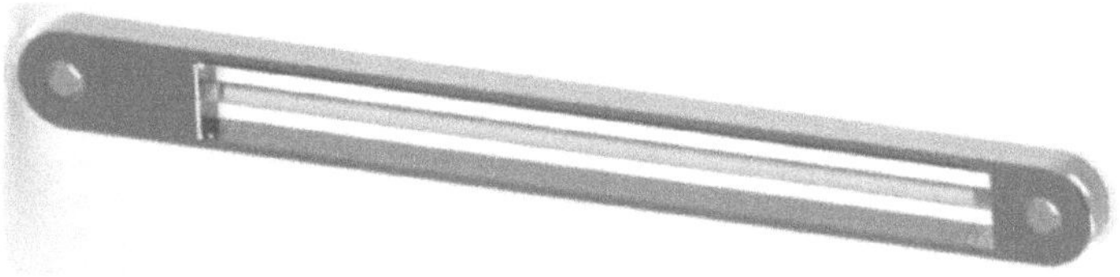

**Figure 4.38** A typical linkage in an SLE structure with movable midspan pins.

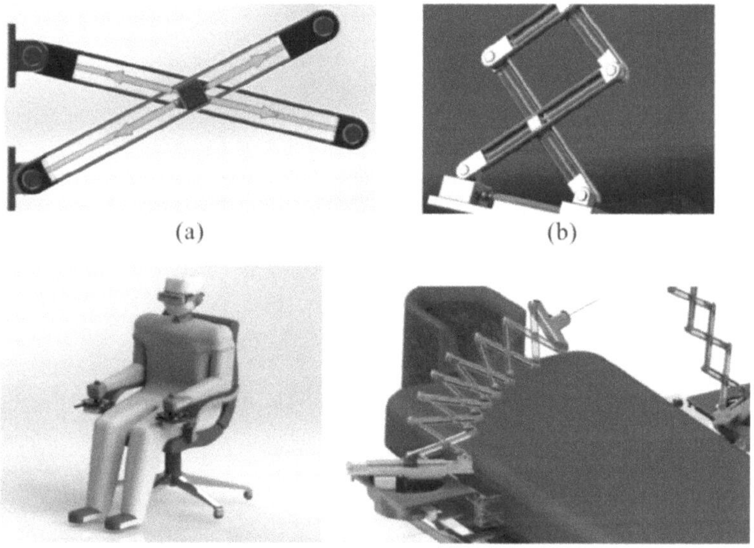

(a) (b)

(c) (d)

**Figure 4.39** The proposed space-efficient robotic surgical system; different views.

Typically four arms are employed to perform robotic surgeries, but depending upon the complexity and need of a surgery, more arms can be utilized. The robotic arms can be either fixed to the sides of a surgical bed or put on a rail in order to be able to slide along the bed to perform surgeries on different parts of the body. As depicted in accompanying diagrams, the body of the structure can be covered with a flexible latex-like tube, preventing contact of human hands with the structure of the robotic system.

Figure 4.40 and 4.41 are views from the surgical scene, with flexible plastic sleeves installed around the deployable structure and covers on double-structure arms, respectively.

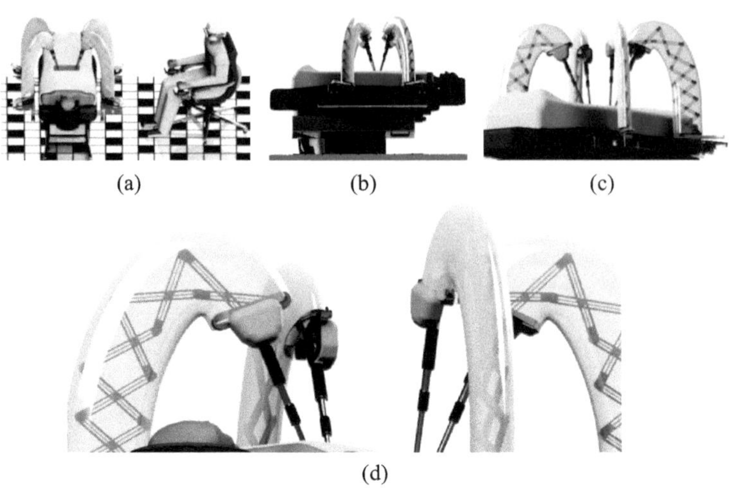


**Figure 4.40** Different views from the surgical scene; flexible tubes installed around the deployable structure.

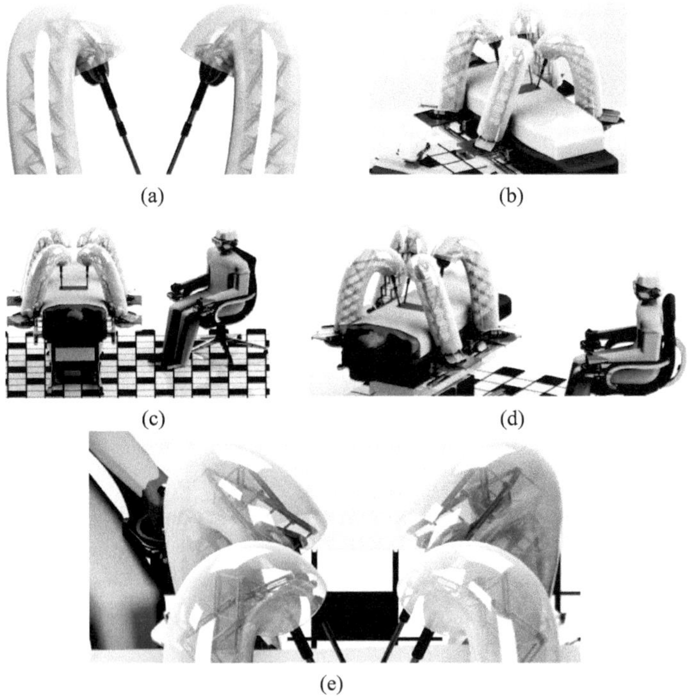


**Figure 4.41** Application of covers on double-structure arms for enhanced safety.

In the proposed surgical system, at least one degree of rotational freedom is considered for surgical instruments. This rotation is about the axis of the surgical instrument, and its associated actuator is installed on the instrument itself.

Redundant safety features can be considered for the robotic surgical system in order to prevent any possible damage to target organs. These features include position limit, speed limit, force limit, etc.

Different actuation methods and mechanisms can be utilized for altering the position of the intermediate pins, that of the first linkage set, and the rotation and tilting of the base. These methods include mechanical, hydraulic, pneumatic, piezoelectric, and electromechanical actuation and the use of parallel mechanisms.

The proposed robotic system is ideal for shipping to places with people in need of medical operations, such as battlefields, as that is one of the major goals of robotic surgery.

### 4.4.2 Forward and Inverse Kinematic Analysis

In the following section we derive forward kinematic equations for the proposed 3D deployable robotic surgical manipulator. Parameters of the robotic surgical arm are shown in Fig. 4.42.

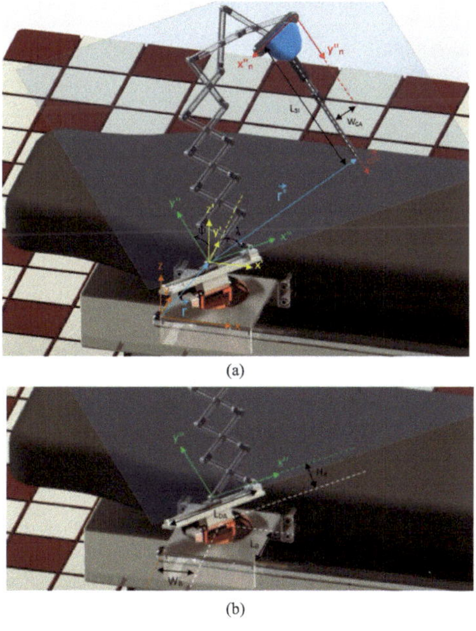

**Figure 4.42** Parameters of the proposed deployable robotic surgical arm.

For the $x''y''$ deployment plane shown in Fig. 4.42, Eq. 4.2 becomes

$$\begin{bmatrix} X'' \\ Y'' \\ 1 \end{bmatrix}_n = \prod_{i=1}^{n} \begin{bmatrix} \cos\theta_{\Delta_i} & -\sin\theta_{\Delta_i} & p_i \\ \sin\theta_{\Delta_i} & \cos\theta_{\Delta_i} & q_i \\ 0 & 0 & 1 \end{bmatrix} . \begin{bmatrix} X''_n \\ Y''_n \\ 1 \end{bmatrix} \tag{4.22}$$

$X''_n$ and $Y''_n$ are the position components of the tip of the surgical instrument in the $x''_n y''_n$ plane:

$X''_n = W_{\text{CA}}$

$Y''_n = L_{\text{SI}}$

Other parameters in Eq. 4.2 remain the same, as defined in Fig. 4.34.

Thus, the position of the tip of the surgical instrument in the $x''y''$ coordinate frame is

$$\mathbf{r}'_{x''y''} = X'' \cdot \mathbf{i}_{x''y''} + Y'' \cdot \mathbf{j}_{x''y''} \tag{4.23}$$

Components of $\mathbf{r}'$ in the $x'y'z'$ coordinate system are

$$\mathrm{r}'_{x'} = X'' \cdot \sin\lambda - Y'' \cdot \sin\theta \cdot \cos\lambda$$

$$\mathrm{r}'_{y'} = X'' \cdot \cos\lambda + Y'' \cdot \sin\theta \cdot \sin\lambda$$

$$\mathrm{r}'_{z'} = Y'' \cdot \cos\theta$$

Thus, $\mathbf{r}'$ in the $x'y'z'$ coordinate system is

$$\begin{aligned} \mathbf{r}'_{x'y'z'} &= (X'' \cdot \sin\lambda - Y'' \cdot \sin\theta \cdot \cos\lambda) \cdot \mathbf{i}_{x'y'z'} \\ &\quad + (X'' \cdot \cos\lambda + Y'' \cdot \sin\theta \cdot \sin\lambda).\mathbf{j}_{x'y'z'} + (Y'' \cdot \cos\theta) \cdot \mathbf{k}_{x'y'z'} \end{aligned} \tag{4.24}$$

or

$$\begin{bmatrix} \mathrm{r}'_{x'} \\ \mathrm{r}'_{y'} \\ \mathrm{r}'_{z'} \end{bmatrix} = \begin{bmatrix} \sin\lambda & -\sin\theta.\cos\lambda & 0 \\ \cos\lambda & \sin\theta.\sin\lambda & 0 \\ 0 & \cos\theta & 0 \end{bmatrix} . \begin{bmatrix} X'' \\ Y'' \\ 1 \end{bmatrix} \tag{4.25}$$

The position of the tip of the surgical instrument in the $xyz$ coordinate frame is

$$\mathbf{r}_{xyz}^{\text{SI tip}} = \mathbf{r}_{xyz} + \mathbf{r'}_{x'y'z'} \tag{4.26}$$

where we have $\mathbf{r}_{x'y'z'}$ and $\mathbf{r}_{xyz}$ calculated as the following:

$$\mathrm{r}_x = W_\mathrm{B} - H_\mathrm{B}\cdot\sin\theta\cdot\cos\lambda + \left(\frac{L_\mathrm{DA}}{2} - c_1\right)\cdot\sin\lambda$$

$$\mathrm{r}_y = L_\mathrm{B} + H_\mathrm{B}\cdot\sin\theta\cdot\sin\lambda + \left(\frac{L_\mathrm{DA}}{2} - c_1\right)\cdot\cos\lambda$$

$$\mathrm{r}_z = H_B\cdot\cos\theta$$

or

$$\begin{aligned}\mathbf{r}_{xyz} = &\left(W_B - H_\mathrm{B}\cdot\sin\theta\cdot\cos\lambda + \left(\frac{L_\mathrm{DA}}{2} - c_1\right)\cdot\sin\lambda\right)\cdot\mathbf{i}_{xyz}\\ &+\left(L_\mathrm{B} + H_\mathrm{B}\cdot\sin\theta\cdot\sin\lambda + \left(\frac{L_\mathrm{DA}}{2} - c_1\right)\cdot\cos\lambda\right)\cdot\mathbf{j}_{xyz} + \left(H_\mathrm{B}\cdot\cos\theta\right)\cdot\mathbf{k}_{xyz}\end{aligned} \tag{4.27}$$

Thus we have

$$\begin{bmatrix}\mathrm{r}_x^{\text{SI tip}}\\ \mathrm{r}_y^{\text{SI tip}}\\ \mathrm{r}_z^{\text{SI tip}}\end{bmatrix} = \begin{bmatrix}\sin\lambda & -\sin\theta\cdot\cos\lambda & 0\\ \cos\lambda & \sin\theta\cdot\sin\lambda & 0\\ 0 & \cos\theta & 0\end{bmatrix} . \begin{bmatrix}X''\\ Y''\\ 1\end{bmatrix} + \begin{bmatrix}W_\mathrm{B} - H_\mathrm{B}\cdot\sin\theta\cdot\cos\lambda + \left(\frac{L_\mathrm{DA}}{2} - c_1\right)\cdot\sin\lambda\\ L_\mathrm{B} + H_\mathrm{B}\cdot\sin\theta\cdot\sin\lambda + \left(\frac{L_\mathrm{DA}}{2} - c_1\right)\cdot\cos\lambda\\ H_\mathrm{B}\cdot\cos\theta\end{bmatrix} \tag{4.28}$$

or in general

$$\begin{bmatrix}\mathrm{r}_x^{\text{SI tip}}\\ \mathrm{r}_y^{\text{SI tip}}\\ \mathrm{r}_z^{\text{SI tip}}\end{bmatrix} = \begin{bmatrix}\sin\lambda & -\sin\theta.\cos\lambda & 0\\ \cos\lambda & \sin\theta.\sin\lambda & 0\\ 0 & \cos\theta & 0\end{bmatrix} . \left(\prod_{i=1}^{n}\begin{bmatrix}\cos\theta_{\Delta_i} & -\sin\theta_{\Delta_i} & p_i\\ \sin\theta_{\Delta_i} & \cos\theta_{\Delta_i} & q_i\\ 0 & 0 & 1\end{bmatrix}\right.\left.\right. . \Bigg[$$

$$\left[\begin{matrix} W_{\mathrm{CA}} \\ L_{\mathrm{SI}} \\ 1 \end{matrix}\right]\Bigg) + \left[\begin{matrix} W_{\mathrm{B}} - H_{\mathrm{B}}.\sin\theta.\cos\lambda + \left(\dfrac{L_{\mathrm{DA}}}{2} - c_1\right).\sin\lambda \\ L_{\mathrm{B}} + H_{\mathrm{B}}.\sin\theta.\sin\lambda + \left(\dfrac{L_{\mathrm{DA}}}{2} - c_1\right).\cos\lambda \\ H_{\mathrm{B}}.\cos\theta \\ \end{matrix}\right] \tag{4.29}$$

$$\mathbf{r}_{xyz}^{\mathrm{SI\,tip}} = \mathrm{r}_x^{\mathrm{SI\,tip}}.\mathbf{i}_{xyz} + \mathrm{r}_y^{\mathrm{SI\,tip}}.\mathbf{j}_{xyz} + \mathrm{r}_z^{\mathrm{SI\,tip}}.\mathbf{k}_{xyz} \tag{4.30}$$

According to Eq. 4.21, the orientation of the surgical instrument in the $x''y''$ plane is

$$\theta_{x''y''}^{\mathrm{inc}} = \text{Total incline in } x''y'' \text{ plane} = \sum_{i=1}^{n-1} \theta_{\Delta_{i+1}}$$

Referring to Fig. 4.42, the components of the unit vector of the direction of the surgical instrument in *xyz* are

$$\mathrm{o}_x^{\mathrm{SI}} = \cos\theta_{x''y''}^{\mathrm{inc}}.\sin\lambda - \sin\theta_{x''y''}^{\mathrm{inc}}.\sin\theta.\cos\lambda$$

$$\mathrm{o}_y^{\mathrm{SI}} = \cos\theta_{x''y''}^{\mathrm{inc}}.\cos\lambda + \sin\theta_{x''y''}^{\mathrm{inc}}.\sin\theta.\sin\lambda$$

$$\mathrm{o}_z^{\mathrm{SI}} = \sin\theta_{x''y''}^{\mathrm{inc}}.\cos\theta$$

Thus

$$\begin{aligned} \mathbf{o}_{xyz}^{\mathrm{SI}} = &\left(\cos\theta_{x''y''}^{\mathrm{inc}}.\sin\lambda - \sin\theta_{x''y''}^{\mathrm{inc}}.\sin\theta.\cos\lambda\right).\mathbf{i}_{xyz} \\ &+ \left(\cos\theta_{x''y''}^{\mathrm{inc}}.\cos\lambda + \sin\theta_{x''y''}^{\mathrm{inc}}.\sin\theta.\sin\lambda\right).\mathbf{j}_{xyz} \\ &+ \left(\sin\theta_{x''y''}^{\mathrm{inc}}.\cos\theta\right).\mathbf{k}_{xyz} \end{aligned} \tag{4.31}$$

The unit vector of the direction of the surgical instrument in *xyz* is

$$\mathbf{e}_{xyz}^{\mathbf{o}^{\mathrm{SI}}} = \frac{\mathbf{o}_{xyz}^{\mathrm{SI}}}{|\,\overrightarrow{\mathbf{o}_{xyz}^{\mathrm{SI}}}\,|} \tag{4.32}$$

The proposed robotic arm can take multiple configurations to deliver a surgical instrument at a specific point at a specific orientation. To find the best configuration, which is inverse kinematics, we need to define an optimization objective. For instance, to move from one configuration to another, we can minimize the sweep area, the electrical energy used by the system, etc. Once the objective is known, we can determine the system parameters with the use of numerical methods since there is no interest in pursuing an analytical solution for such complex forward kinematics equations. Determining a reasonable optimization objective requires more study and is not covered in this book.

## Problem Set

1. Describe laparoscopic and robotic laparoscopic surgery.
2. What are the two frequent approaches to perform minimally invasive surgeries with the help of robots? Describe them.
3. What units is a teleoperative robotic system comprised of? Describe them.
4. What were/are the first methods and systems in robotic laparoscopy? Describe them.
5. What is the difference between the conventional laparoscopy and robotic laparoscopy? You can use da Vinci surgical system as an example.
6. What are the five main units any robot-assisted surgical system is comprised of?
7. What is "dual console capability"?
8. Describe da Vinci® EndoWrist® instruments.
9. What are cannulas?
10. What are smart deployable structures?
11. What are SLE structures, and what are their advantages?
12. Describe how the proposed space-saving surgical system for use in laparoscopy was conceived and developed.
13. Describe the major units of the proposed space-saving laparoscopic robotic surgical system.
14. What are the degrees of freedom of the proposed surgical system?
15. Generate the 3D workspace of the developed surgical system using the derived equations in Chapter 4.
16. Generate the motion trajectory of the tip of the surgical instrument using the equations derived in Chapter 4 with a number of arbitrary set of constraints.

Chapter 5

# Applications of Smart Materials and Artificial Muscles in Robotic Surgery

## 5.1 Introduction to Smart Materials and Artificial Muscles

In this chapter we will introduce a number of smart materials and artificial muscles that can be employed during robotic surgery to enhance the quality of surgical operations with robotic structures and provide force, haptic, and kinesthetic feedback to surgeons during robotic surgery. Smart materials are generally defined as multifunctional materials that can perform sensing, energy harvesting, and actuation, in addition to providing additional signals pertaining to their environmental disturbances and changes. Due to the requirement of biocompatibility, not all smart materials can be easily used in robotic surgery. For example, piezoceramic materials such as lead zirconate titanate (PZT) are not recommended for use in a biomedical environment due to the presence of lead-related materials. However, piezopolymeric materials such as polyvinylidene fluoride (PVDFT) may be used. Here we introduce biomimetic ionic polymer metal composites (IPMCs) as electroactive polymers (EAPs) and artificial muscles, conductive and conjugated polymers, metal hydride artificial muscles, chemoelectromechanical contractile

*Robotic Surgery: Smart Materials, Robotic Structures, and Artificial Muscles*
Mohsen Shahinpoor and Siavash Gheshmi

ISBN 978-981-4316-23-1 (Hardcover), 978-981-4463-51-5 (eBook)
www.panstanford.com

artificial muscles such as polyascrylonitrile fibrous gels (PAN gels), biopolymeric artificial muscles such as chitosan gels, magnetic gels, shape memory alloys (SMAs), and shape memory polymers (SMPs) to robotic surgery and discuss possible applications of other multifunctional smart materials and artificial muscles in robotic surgery. For a comprehensive reference on intelligent materials see Shahinpoor and Schneider (2008). For a reference on artificial muscles see Shahinpoor (2002) and Shahinpoor, Kim, and Mojarrad (2007).

## 5.2 Applications of Ionic Polymer Metal Composites in Robotic Surgery

### 5.2.1 Brief Introduction to IPMCs as Multifunctional Materials

IPMCs, or ionic polymer conductor nanocomposites (IPCNCs), are chemically plated ionic polymers manufactured by oxidation-reduction (REDOX) operations with a noble metal, such as platinum or gold, to keep them biocompatible. Refer to a seminal publication by Shahinpoor, Kim, and Mojarrad (2007) for a comprehensive coverage of various properties and applications of such materials. For more information on modeling of IPMCs see Shahinpoor (2000), de Gennes, Okumura, Shahinpoor, and Kim (2002), Shahinpoor (2003, 2005, 2008 and 2009) and Shahinpoor and Kim (2002). For information on manufacturing IPMCs see Shahinpoor, Kim, and Mojarrad (2007) and Kim and Shahinpoor (2005). For medical and industrial applications of IPMCs see Shahinpoor and Kim (2005). The basic material is commonly ionic Teflon with relatively few fixed ionic groups. Once an electric field is imposed on such a network, the conjugated and hydrated cations rearrange to accommodate the local electric field, and thus the network deforms, and in the simplest of cases such as in thin-membrane sheets, spectacular bending is observed (Fig. 5.1) under small electric fields such as tens of volts per millimeter.

Typical experimental deflection curves are depicted below in Figs. 5.2 and 5.3.

Once an electric field is imposed on an IPMC cantilever, in the cantilever polymeric network the hydrated cations migrate to accommodate the local electric field. This creates a pressure gradient across the thickness of the beam, and thus the beam undergoes bending deformation (Fig. 5.4) under small electric fields such as tens of volts per millimeter. Figure 5.4 depicts typical force and deflection characteristics of cantilever samples of ionic polymer metal nanocomposite (IPMNC) artificial muscles.

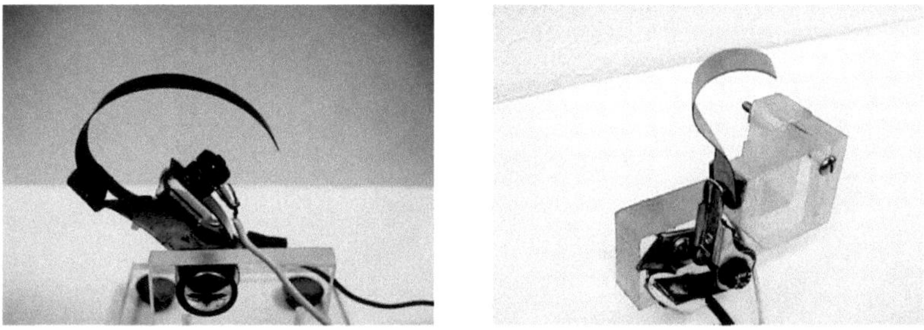

**Figure 5.1** Typical deformation of strips (10 × 80 × 0.34 mm) of ionic polymers under a step voltage of 4 V.

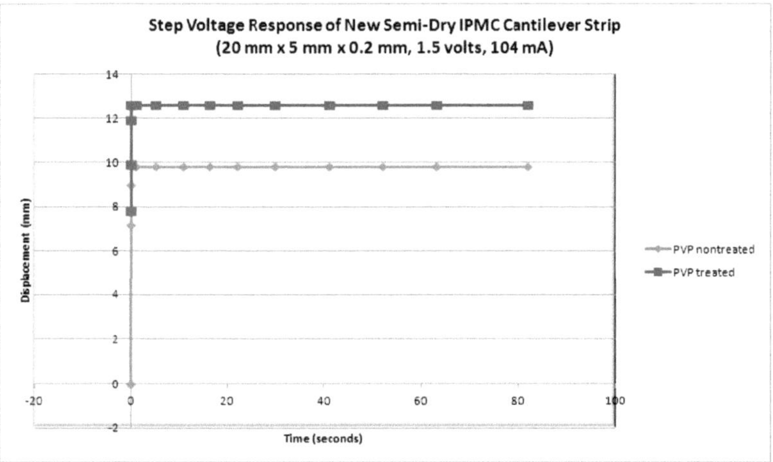


**Figure 5.2** Step response displacement characteristics of IPMNC samples ($\delta$: arc length, $L_o$: effective beam length). $L_o$ = 1.5 inches (bottom).

IPMCs can generate electrical power like an electromechanical battery if flexed, bent, twisted, torsioned, or squeezed. Keshavarzi, Shahinpoor, Kim and Lantz (1999) applied the transduction capability of IPMCs to the measurement of blood pressure, pulse rate, and rhythm measurement using thin sheets of IPMCs during surgery. Motivated by the idea of measuring pressure in the human spine, Ferrara, et al. (1999) applied pressure across the thickness of an IPMC strip while measuring the output voltage. Typically, flexing of such material in cantilever form sets it into a damped vibration mode that can generate a similar damped signal in the form of electrical power (voltage or current), as shown in Fig. 5.5.

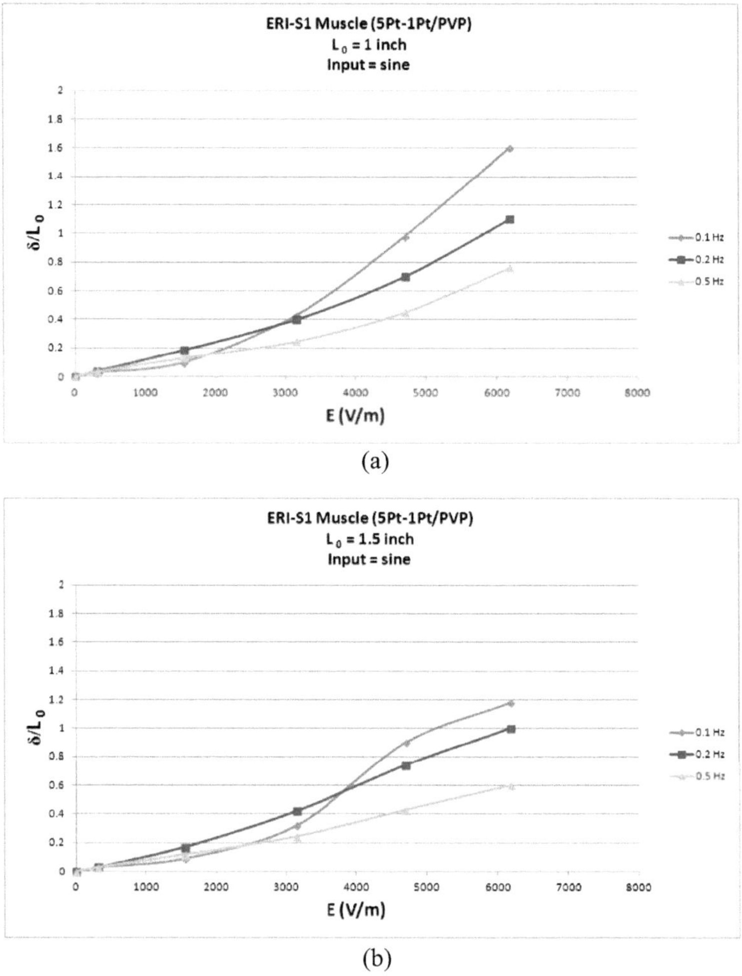


**Figure 5.3** Displacement characteristics of an IPMC, ERI-S1 ($\delta$: arc length, $L_0$: effective cantilever beam length). $L_0$ = 1 inch (top, a) and 1.5 inches (bottom, b).

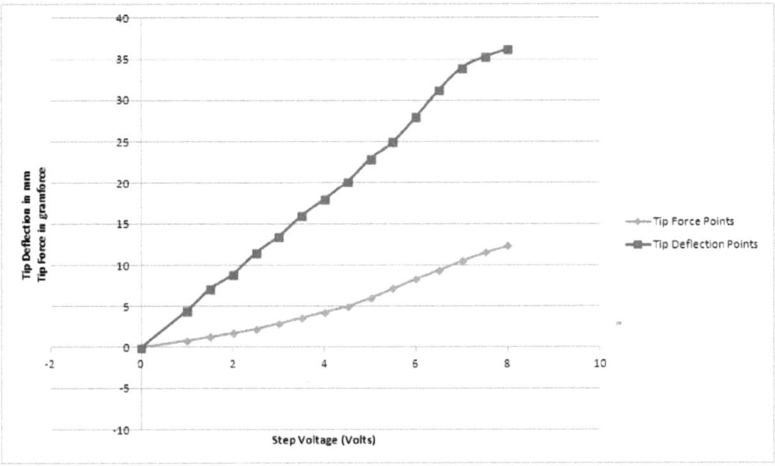


**Figure 5.4** Variation of tip-blocking force and the associated deflection if allowed to move vs. the applied step voltage for a 1 cm × 5 cm × 0.3 mm IPMNC Pt-Pd sample in a cantilever configuration.

The experimental results showed that almost a linear relationship exists between the voltage output and the imposed displacement of the tip of the IPMNC sensor. As far as force generation is concerned, IPMNCs generally have a very high force. Figure 5.6 below displays the cantilever and load cell configuration for measuring the tip-blocking force of typical samples of IPMNCs.

## 5.3 Feasibility of Providing Kinesthetic Force Feedback to Surgeons during Robotic Surgery by Electroactive Polymeric Sensors

One can integrate IPMCs as electroactive polymeric nanosensors and nanoactuators with robotic surgical end effectors such as intuitive grasping forceps to provide kinesthetic force/torque feedback to surgeons during robotic surgery. The application is to employ IPMCs as surgeons' feel/haptic sensors for the kinesthetics of internal organs in interaction with various surgical robotic end effectors. The application is to integrate the kinesthetic force feedback signals with joysticks and foot pedals for surgeons to receive kinesthetic force feedback, on the fly, during robotic surgery.

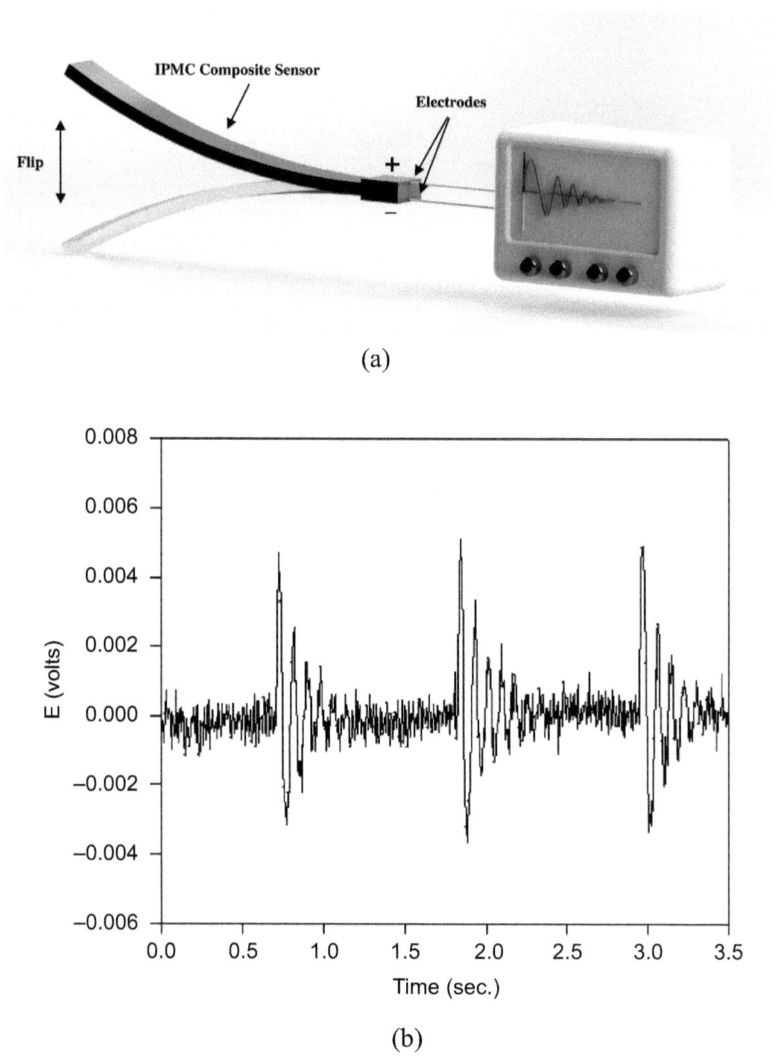


**Figure 5.5** A typical voltage response of an IPMC strip (1 cm × 4 cm × 0.2 mm) under oscillatory mechanical excitations. (a) Setup of cantilever configuration and (b) dynamic voltage output.

In achieving these objectives suitable IPMC strips and loops are attached to the end effectors and wired through the end effectors to the electronics providing kinesthetic force or torque feedback to surgeons. To provide that force or torque sensation to the surgeons, the specific IPMC sensor, say a tip bender, will be subjected to a bending force to create an output signal in millivolts. This signal will then be amplified electronically and fed into a linear actuator or servo motor to generate the same force or torque and affect the operational forces/torques in the joysticks or foot pedals used by surgeons. If the tip of a 3 cm × 1 cm × 0.2 mm IPMC strip experiences a blocking force by contacting an organ/tissue during surgery it will develop a blocking kinesthetic force of about 20 g. The same strip in a cantilever configuration if moved by the kinesthetics of internal organs and end effectors during surgery will generate about 4 mV, which can be correlated to the kinesthetic forces of the internal organ movement during robotic surgery. Our experimentally obtained data indicates that IPMCs may provide a dynamic feedback of kinesthetic forces to the surgeons during surgery and gradually train surgeons to feel out the kinesthetics and kinesthetic forces and torques applied to internal organs and tissues during surgery.

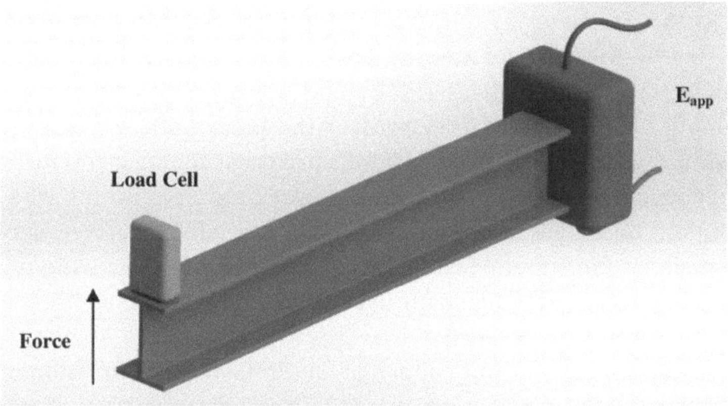


**Figure 5.6** Cantilever and load cell configuration for measuring the tip-blocking force of IPMNC samples.

The fact that IPMCs can work well in the wet human body environment during robotic surgery will be an advantage for developing this technology. IPMCs are basically biocompatible because they are Teflon-based plastics in a nanocomposite form with a noble metal, such as platinum or gold. They are electrically safe and self-powered and do not need any source of voltage or current to provide kinesthetic force feedback in millivolts, and they are autoclaveable and hardly wear out. IPMCs also work well in an electrocautery environment because IPMCs are basically ionic Teflon with platinum electrodes that can withstand the high temperature of cauterization without melting or burning during surgery.

The current robotic surgical systems evolved from laparoscopic surgical procedures and made it possible for surgeons to perform surgery away from the patient with much more concentration and ease. However, what was lost in this transition by the surgeons was the feeling sensation of tissues and organs and kinesthetic force feedback during surgery. It is interesting to note that even during laparoscopic surgery the surgeons can still feel and sense the tissues and organs they are handling and operating on with laparoscopic/endoscopic tools and feel the kinesthetic forces at work. However, kinesthetic force feedback was replaced with visual feedback during robotic surgery.

It is to be noted that some of this kinesthetic force feedback was lost in the transition from open to laparoscopic surgery due to trocar friction and varying lever arms, anyway. However, with smart materials such as IPMCs and appropriate calibration and tuning one may be able to recover the kinesthetic force feedback during surgery using IPMCs. IPMCs are great for such robotic force feedback applications because they work perfectly well in the wet human body environment and generate millivolt-level sensing signals for kinesthetic force feedback. Figure 5.7 depicts the typical sensing output of IPMC strips in bending and how the bending force is measured by a load cell.

Note that the output voltage of an IPMC strip is a function of the curvature and its rate of change. While an output voltage of 1-2 mV can be derived by dynamic sensing from a sample with dimensions of 10 mm × 30 mm × 0.2 mm, the achievable voltage is smaller in quasi-static sensing case using the same sample.

An IPMC generates signals in the range of a few millivolts in the presence of deformation. IPMC sensors have proven to be highly sensitive to the applied deformation over a large frequency range. Figure 5.8 shows the general response of an IPMC sensor to fast excitations followed by slow bending accompanied with high-frequency noise.

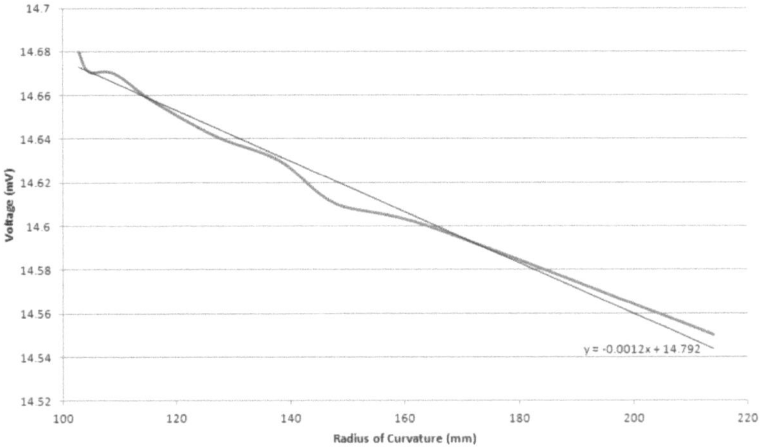


**Figure 5.7** Typical sensing response of IPMC strips in bending. The sensing response is in millivolts, which can be correlated to the tip kinesthetic force

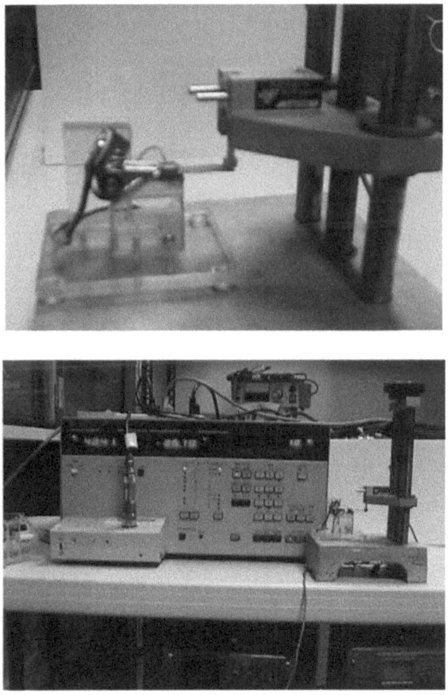

**Figure 5.8** Experimental set-up for the measurement of bending force and curvature of IPMC cantilever strips using a high resolution load cell and impedance analyzer.

To obtain kinesthetic force feedback information from IPMCs, two calibration procedures are required. To this end the calibration of deformation of an IPMC sensor with respect to the generated signal and then the bending force of an IPMC actuator can be easily related to the observed deformation. It should be emphasized that the results of using IPMCs as kinesthetic force feedback to surgeons during robotic surgery are very promising in that kinesthetic force feedback to surgeons may be possible using IPMCs in bending, twisting, loop, or compression loading. In the next section we will elaborate on some additional experimental data that may help achieve our objectives.

## 5.4 Integration of IPMCs with Robotic End Effectors for Kinesthetic Force Feedback to Surgeons during Robotic Surgery by Electroactive Polymeric Sensors

IPMCs with distributed nanosensing and nanoactuation can be employed in robotic surgery in order to provide kinesthetic force feedback to surgeons. Several apparatuses for modeling and testing of the various IPMC artificial muscles are described to show the viability of the application of electroactive IPMCs for providing surgeons with kinesthetic force feedback during robotic surgery. Here we present some of the data generated by placing small strips of IPMCs on the contact face of grasping forceps, as shown in Fig. 5.9 below.

One can also explore the bending and loop configurations for IPMCs (Fig. 5.10) to interact with bodily organs and tissues during robotic surgery and provide kinesthetic force signals due to bending of the IPMC strips or deformation of the loop, which provides a voltage signal that can be correlated to the force exerted.

Kinesthetic force feedback signals in the range of a few millivolts can be generated by touching soft plastic organs and can be correlated with the grasping forces by surgeons. Figures 5.11, 5.12, and 5.13 show some typical sensing signals out of IPMC strips attached to surgical robotic end effectors in compression, bending, and loop configurations.

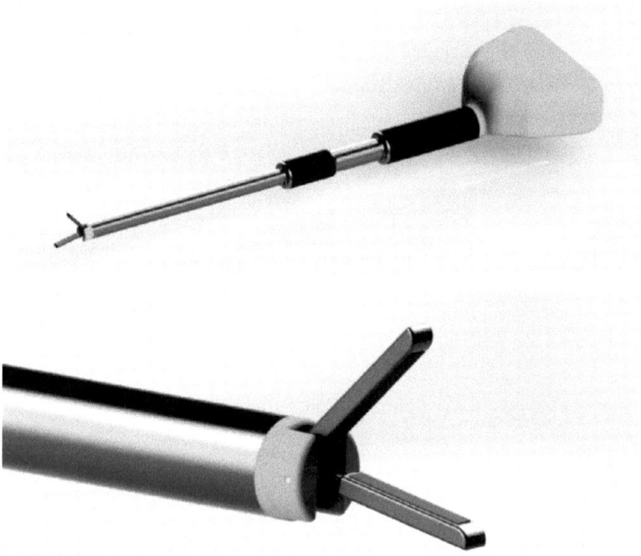

**Figure 5.9** IPMC strips mounted on the face of grasping forceps (top and bottom) and wired in to the electronics.

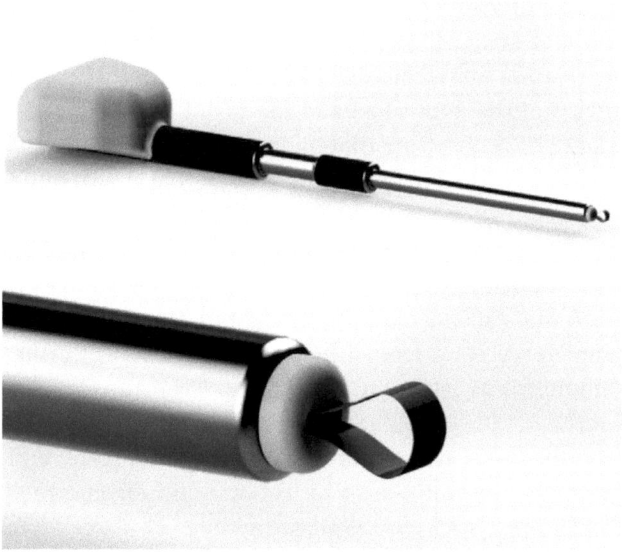

**Figure 5.10** Kinesthetic force feedback loop for haptic interaction with bodily organs.

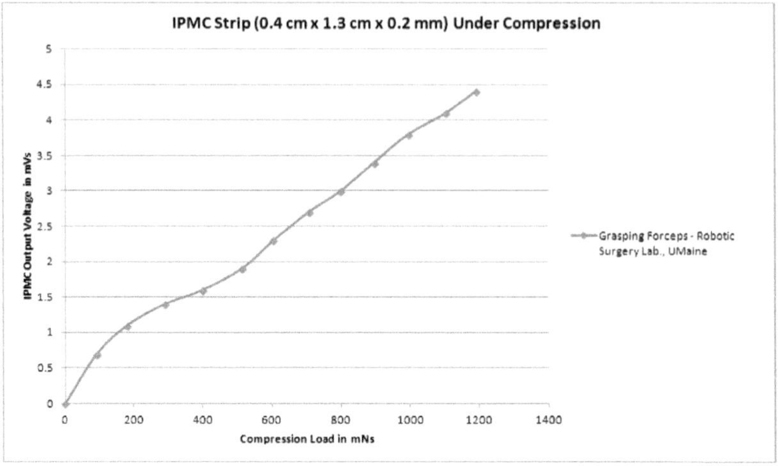


**Figure 5.11** Typical strong sensing signal in millivolts out of an IPMC strip in compression mode (direct compression of IPMCs with a normal load).

By compression we mean direct compression of IPMCs with a normal load such as in grasping forceps (Fig. 5.14). Note that the voltage output can be correlated with kinesthetic normal force applied to the strip, electronically, as described below.

The relation between the bending moment $M$ and radius of curvature $\rho$ of the neutral axis of the beam is as follows: $M = EI/\rho$, where $I = (1/12)\ \mathrm{bh}^3$. Note that on the basis of the dimensions given in Fig. 5.7 (10 × 30 × 0.2 mm), $I = (1/12) \times (0.01) \times (0.0002)^3 = 6.67 \times 10^{-15}\ \mathrm{m}^4$, and with $E = 1200$ MPa for IPMCs and considering pure bending, we can calculate the required force for bending: $F = M/L = M/0.03 = 33.3M$. Thus on the basis of the curvatures measured in Fig. 5.7, one can calculate the corresponding $M$ and calculate the equivalent force experienced by bending an IPMC during surgery. For example, for $\rho = 100$ mm, $M = 81 \times 10^{-6}$ Nm and $F = 2.74 \times 10^{-3}$ N = 2.74 mN.

Thus, to make robotic surgery more intelligent and haptics based one should equip surgical robotic end effectors with smart nanocomposites such as IPMCs capable of force, haptic, and impedance sensing that can be fed back to the surgeon. Thus, one will be able to correlate the signal out of the IPMC mounted on an end effector to the kinesthetic force experienced by the IPMC strip.

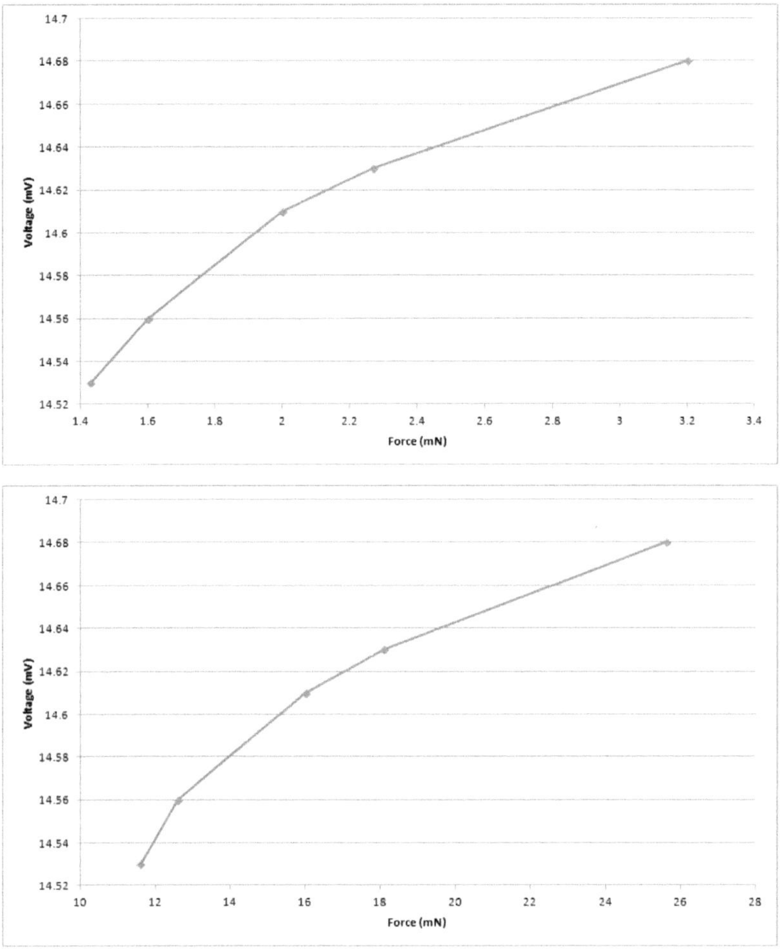


**Figure 5.12** Typical force sensing signal in milli-Newton out of an IPMC strip (top: 10 × 30 × 0.2 mm, bottom: 10 × 30 × 0.4 mm) in bending/twisting mode (bending or twisting of IPMCs due to kinesthetic interaction).

To translate the kinesthetic force feedback voltage signal from the IPMC strips to kinesthetic force feedback to the surgeon's hands during surgery, the voltage signal will be amplified electronically and applied to a servo motor integrated with joysticks to simultaneously provide the surgeon with kinesthetic force feedback. For other kinesthetic configurations of IPMCs, such as bending kinesthetic or loop kinesthetic, similar operations are applied. Figure 5.15 depicts the general experimental setup to correlate the sensing voltage signal coming off the bending or loop configurations of IPMCs in kinesthetic interaction with end effectors and organs with the actual kinesthetic forces at work in Newton.

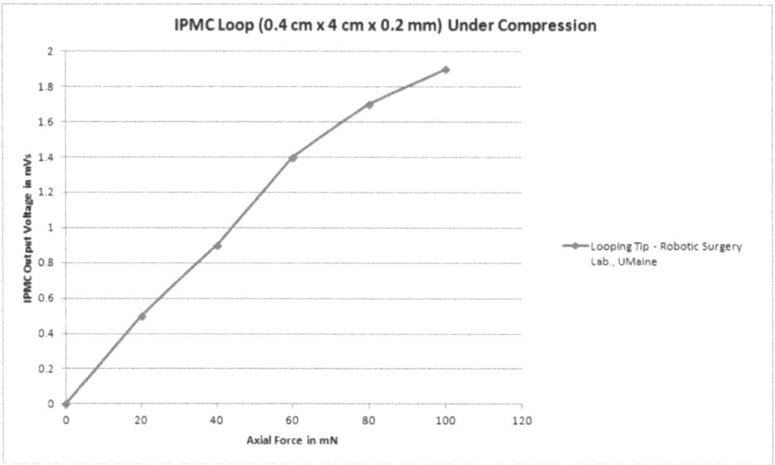


**Figure 5.13** Typical sensing signal in millivolts out of an IPMC in a loop configuration (loop deformation of IPMCs due to kinesthetic interaction of da Vinci® end effectors and plastic body organs). The voltage output can be correlated with kinesthetic normal force applied to the strip.

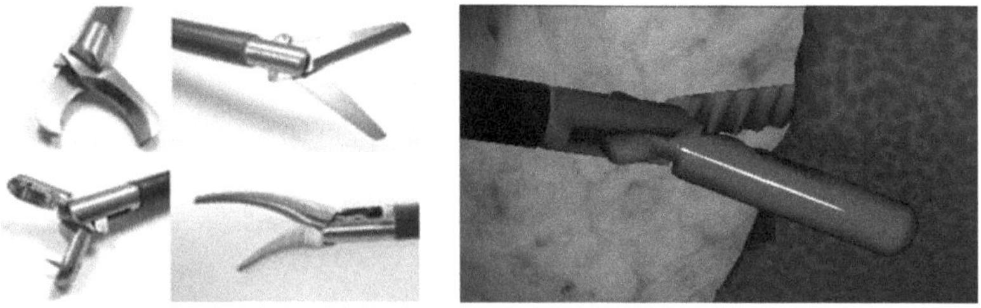

**Figure 5.14** Some of typical da Vinci® surgical end effectors that can be integrated with various configuration of IPMCs for sensing the contact surfaces and kinesthetic forces experienced by surgeons during robotic surgery.

The IPMC bending sensor is attached to a cantilever beam so that the IPMC strip follows the imposed curvature of the beam shape.

One end of the sample is clamped to the fixed end of the beam. Both curvature and the rate of change of curvature are controlled using a servo motor, which bends the tip of the beam. An AX-12 Dynamixel servo motor with a step size of 0.29° was used to control the tip bending of the cantilever beam. The servo motor is also controlled through LabVIEW software. For voltage measurement, an NI-9219 A/D data acquisition module was used, and the data was processed in LabVIEW. To reduce the signal noise, a band pass filter was used to filter low (below 0.01 Hz) and high (higher than 5 Hz) frequencies. The output voltage was amplified by a factor of 10 for easier processing of data. To calibrate the sensor, different curvature inputs were applied to the cantilever at different rates.

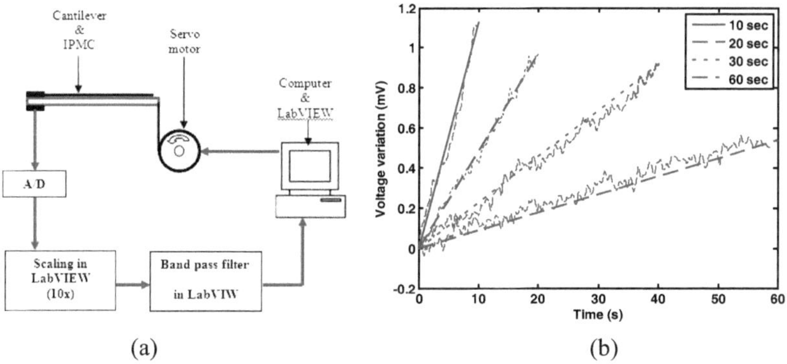


**Figure 5.15** (a) Schematic of the experimental setup to measure the dynamic kinesthetic output voltage of IPMC strips in bending and electronically correlate it to the forces generated via torque measurements of the servo motor. (b) Ramp response of an IPMC sensor at four different curvature rates of 10 seconds, 20 seconds, 40 seconds, and 60 seconds. The IPMC strip was dynamically bent for an amount of 10 mm, which is equal to a 500 mm radius of curvature.

Incorporating haptic force feedback may also enable expansion of robotic surgery to other surgical procedures, such as intraocular surgery or microsurgery, that are difficult to perform without a sense of touch or force feedback integrated with surgical robotic end effectors. These robotic end effectors, such as needle holders, grasping forceps, dissecting forceps, scissors, biopsy spoons, retractors, electrosurgical tips, and retractors and uterine manipulators, play a fundamental role in robotic surgery. IPMCs can also be made as microgripper for microsurgery applications such as ophthalmic surgery. For a reference on IPMC microgrippers see Deole et al. (2008).

## Problem Set

1. Describe how IPMCs can be used in laparoscopic and robotic laparoscopic surgery.
2. What are the two frequent approaches to perform minimally invasive surgeries with the help of robots equipped with artificial muscles? Describe them.
3. Why are multifunctional materials important in robotic surgery?
4. What information are IPMCs as soft sensors and actuators used to provide surgeons during robotic surgery?
5. What is the significance of haptic sensing in robotic surgery?
6. What is the significance of tactile sensing of internal body organs during robotic surgery?
7. What is the significance of kinesthetic sensing during robotic surgery?
8. What is the significance and importance of force feedback to surgeons during robotic surgery?
9. How could smart materials be integrated with robotic surgery end effectors? Describe a number of possibilities and configurations.
10. Describe a scenario for experimental measurement of dynamic kinesthetic output voltage of IPMCs for application to robotic surgery.
11. How could the output voltage obtained in the previous problem be electronically correlated to the forces applied or experienced by bodily organs during robotic surgery?
12. How can forces applied to bodily organs be translated in terms of the forces or torques in joysticks operated by surgeons during robotic surgery?
13. How could the fact that IPMCs do respond differently (generate different voltages, depending on the rate of loading, bending, or deforming) be used to give more force and haptic feedback to surgeons?

# Chapter 6

# Summary and Conclusions

In Chapter 1, a brief history of robotics was given and the laws of robotics were introduced. This was followed by an introduction to robotic surgery where the work of several researchers was discussed. The advantages of robotic surgical systems were expounded, and finally, different robots for several surgical procedures were introduced.

In Chapter 2, the science of motion of robotic links, regardless of the forces that generate the motion, was introduced. This is commonly known as kinematics of multiaxes robotic structures. This knowledge was then applied to robotic manipulators and objects to be manipulated. First, the structure of a typical multilink or multiaxes robotic manipulator was described and some mathematical notations to be used were introduced. Second, we discussed the applications of $4 \times 4$ and $n \times 4$ homogenous transformations in robotic kinematics. Subsequently, these transformations were used to describe the general position and orientation, that is, the kinematic attitude, of one robotic link with respect to an adjacent robotic link. Thus, the notion of Denavit–Hartenberg (D–H) homogenous transformations was introduced and pertinent equations were derived. Then the concepts of direct kinematics and inverse kinematics were introduced. Finally, the workspace of a robotic manipulator was defined and illustrated for 2D and 3D two-link robotic manipulators.

*Robotic Surgery: Smart Materials, Robotic Structures, and Artificial Muscles*
Mohsen Shahinpoor and Siavash Gheshmi

ISBN 978-981-4316-23-1 (Hardcover), 978-981-4463-51-5 (eBook)
www.panstanford.com

In Chapter 3, ophthalmic surgery was introduced and different types of intraocular surgeries were discussed. This was followed by an introduction to relevant work from different researchers and some robotic surgical systems for use in intraocular surgeries. Our proposed robotic system for ophthalmic surgeries was discussed and its different parts expounded. The core idea behind the design of the proposed surgical system is that intraocular surgical instruments are inserted into the eye from its periphery. Described is a robotic surgical system accordingly with a ring-shaped surgical headmaster around which the robotic manipulators rotate to deliver surgical instruments to the periphery of the eye. This was followed by a kinematics analysis of the robotic system with the help of D–H transformation matrices. Finally, the feasibility of using the proposed system in cataract surgery was studied.

The described intraocular robotic system is composed of two fundamental units, a master surgeon console/station and a robotic surgical slave.

- Master surgeon console: The surgeon's station consists of an ergonomically designed chair, a pair of vision goggles, and a pair of multiple-degrees-of-freedom joysticks. The joysticks can be installed on the chair with the help of two platforms. The imaging goggles generate a panoramic view of the surgical scene and help the microsurgeon maintain a natural posture and handle surgeries more easily and comfortably. Imaging features such as magnification further help the microsurgeon operate more precisely. The surgeon sits on the chair as the master of the robotic surgical procedure and controls the surgical operation via the joysticks. His/her hand movements are scaled, filtered, and translated into movements of surgical instruments snapped onto the robotic slave arms. Using a pair of joysticks and a pair of vision goggles is a space-efficient alternative for bulky robotic surgery operations.
- Robotic surgical slave: The surgical slave robot actually performs the surgery on a patient's eye. It is composed of five main entities: a pedestal, a telescopic tower, a surgical headmaster, robotic arms, and an instrument holder. The pedestal is vibration-isolated, which can be securely locked in place. It moves the telescopic tower horizontally to the left

and right to place the surgical headmaster above the right eye. The telescopic tower moves the surgical headmaster vertically up and down to position it at an appropriate height with respect to the patient's head. The surgical headmaster can also be moved horizontally in a telescopic manner to the front and back for further adjustment in the horizontal plane. It is placed at the right position in the *xyz* telescopic fashion. The headmaster consists of an assembly of cylindrical precision head gears to which a fixed camera, a movable camera, and two or more movable precision multiple-axes robotic manipulators are attached. The fixed camera provides a top view of the surgical operation, while the movable camera rotates around the surgical headmaster to provide a peripheral view of the surgery. The movable camera is attached to a linear actuator, which can adjust its height. A rotary joint also changes its view angle. The two or more robotic manipulators revolve around the surgical headmaster to deliver precision surgical instruments from the periphery of the eye. Each robotic manipulator includes six main units: the base of the arm, a linear actuator in the base of the arm, a base rotary joint, an upper linear actuator, an elbow rotary joint, and a lower linear actuator. The base of the arm rotates the arms around the surgical headmaster. The linear actuator in the base of the arm moves the robotic arms in the radial direction. The base rotary joint rotates the robotic manipulator around the vertical axis of the upper linear actuator. The upper linear actuator and lower linear actuator change their length to manipulate surgical instruments. The elbow rotary joint adjusts the angle between the upper linear actuator and the lower linear actuator. The instrument holder holds the surgical instrument necessary in an operation for the robotic manipulators to pick them up. The instrument holder is in the workspace of the slave robot, and the robotic arms can easily pick any of the surgical instruments. The robotic end effectors are equipped with haptic feedback sensors and force and optical sensors, which help detect forces or disturbances experienced by the robotic end effectors by engagement with the anatomy of the eye. All robotic movements and operations of the manipulator arms, end effectors, the headmaster, and cameras are controlled by the master surgeon from the first major unit, the surgical master station.

Some future work in this area would be:

1. Optimization of the size of the proposed system. This could be done by placing the pedestal on the surgical bed, which results in a much smaller telescopic tower. The diameter of the surgical headmaster can be decreased by considering a captive linear actuator for the lower linear actuators of the robotic manipulators. The linear actuator must not have any rotation at the tip.
2. A parallel mechanism can be used with the upper linear actuators in order to alter the elbow angle of the robotic manipulators. This change will increase precision at the joint.
3. Design for manufacturing.
4. Multibody dynamics and control analysis.
5. Structural analysis.
6. Fabrication.

In Chapter 4, laparoscopic robotic surgery was introduced and the benefits of robotic laparoscopic surgical operations were discussed. This was followed by an introduction to relevant work from different researchers. Then, current systems in robotic laparoscopic surgeries were introduced and expanded upon. Different sections of any robotic surgical system, surgeon console, image processing equipment, surgical instruments, slave robot, and endoscopic camera were introduced. Also introduced were new surgical systems as alternatives to sections one and four of current available surgical robots, surgeon consoles, and slave robots. The core of the proposed surgical system was around using 2D scissor-like element (SLE) structures with servo-motorized midspan pins on a spherical base joint. This configuration yields a highly dexterous robotic system that can operate in 3D. An introduction to deployable structures was given, which included mathematical modeling of these structures, simulation, etc. Our system was then presented and discussed. Finally, the forward and inverse kinematics of the proposed robotic system with complex morphology were discussed.

Our proposed laparoscopic robotic surgical system consists of two major units, a master surgeon console/station and a robotic surgical slave:

- The master surgeon console is the same as the console described for the proposed intraocular robotic system.
- The robotic surgical slave arm is an SLE structure with movable midspan pins that is mounted on a spherical actuator to change its deployment plane. The relative locations of intermediate pins are altered by servo motors located inside linkages. Several of these robotic arms can be attached to the sides of a surgical bed in order to manipulate surgical instruments and endoscopic cameras. At the end of the surgery, the manipulator arms are contracted and can be placed underneath the surgical bed. Movements of these manipulator arms are under direct control of the surgeon as the master of the surgical intervention. With the proposed robotic surgical slave arms, minimal space is taken up in the surgical room during and after operations. Furthermore, the proposed system makes it possible to deploy portable surgical robots in different fields and working areas. Developing portable surgical robots is an important vision for the future of minimally invasive surgery, which will have an impact on a wide variety of applications, from battlefields to space stations.

Some future work in this area would be:

1. The consecutive link sets can be designed in parallel planes in an inward fashion so the whole structure tapers from the base to the tip of the robot. This method yields an even more space-efficient mechanism. In this case, after contraction, the manipulator is converted into a plate. Therefore, the whole robotic arm looks like a thick plate in a closed shape.
2. Further study can be made of the use of non-servo-motorized link sets among servo-motorized ones and how these can affect the kinematic attitude of the robotic system.
3. An optimization objective can be determined on the basis of which the robot can choose any of the redundant configurations to accomplish a specific task.
4. Parallel mechanisms can be used to alter the two rotational variables of the spherical base of the robot. This makes the robotic system robust.
5. Design for manufacturing.

6. Multibody dynamics and control analysis.
7. Structural analysis.

Chapter 5 finally discussed how smart materials can be integrated with surgical robotics end effectors to provide haptic, tactile, force, and kinesthetic feedback from surgical contacts and interaction between the tip of the end effectors, which are mostly surgical instruments such as parallel jaw grippers to suturing structures or feeding suturing threads. The intent of Chapter 5 is to address more advanced surgical operation in which the surgical robotic end effectors are integrated with ionic polymer metal composites (IPMCs). It was noted in Chapter 5 that robotic surgical systems evolved from the laparoscopic surgical procedures and made it possible for surgeons to perform surgery away from the patient with much more concentration and ease. However, what was lost in this transition by the surgeons was the feeling sensation of tissues and organs and kinesthetic force feedback during surgery. It is interesting to note that even during laparoscopic surgery, the surgeons can still feel and sense the tissues and organs they are handling and operating on with laparoscopic/endoscopic tools during surgery and feel the kinesthetic forces at work. However, kinesthetic force feedback was replaced with visual feedback during robotic surgery. It is to be noted that some of this kinesthetic force feedback was lost in the transition from open to laparoscopic surgery due to trocar friction and varying lever arms, anyway. However, with smart materials such as IPMCs and appropriate calibration and tuning one may be able to recover the kinesthetic force feedback during surgery using IPMCs. IPMCs are great for such robotic force feedback applications because they work perfectly well in the wet human body environment and generate millivolt-level sensing signals for kinesthetic force feedback.

# Appendix A

# MATLAB Codes for the Generated Diagrams in Chapter 2

**Fig. 2.16**

```
l1=40;
l2=15;
for theta1=0:0.1:90
    for theta2=0:0.1:90
        x=l1*cosd(theta1)+l2*cosd(theta1+theta2);
    y=l1*sind(theta1)+l2*sind(theta1+theta2);
    plot(x,y,'g.');
    hold on;
    end
end
```

**Fig. 2.17**

```
l1=40;
l2=15;
for theta1=0:0.1:270
    fortheta2=0:0.1:90
        x=l1*cosd(theta1)+l2*cosd(theta1+theta2);
    y=l1*sind(theta1)+l2*sind(theta1+theta2);
    plot(x,y,'g.');
        hold on;
    end
end
```

**Fig. 2.18**

```
l1=40;
l2=15;
l3=5;
for theta1=0:0.1:180
    for theta2=0:0.1:90
        for theta3=0:0.1:90
            x=l1*cosd(theta1)+l2*cosd(theta1+theta2)+
                l3*cosd(theta1+theta2+theta3);
            y=l1*sind(theta1)+l2*sind(theta1+theta2)
                +l3*sind(theta1+theta2+theta3);
            plot(x,y,'b.');
        hold on;
        end
    end
end
```

**Fig. 2.19**

```
l1=40;
l2=15;
l3=5;
fortheta1=0:0.1:90
    for theta2=0:0.1:90
        for theta3=0:0.1:90
            x=l1*cosd(theta1)+l2*cosd(theta1+theta2)+
                l3*cosd(theta1+theta2+theta3);
            y=l1*sind(theta1)+l2*sind(theta1+theta2)+
                l3*sind(theta1+theta2+theta3);
        plot(x,y,'b.');
        hold on;
        end
    end
end
```

**Fig. 2.20**

```
l1=40;
l2=15;
l3=5;
l4=5;
for theta1=0:0.1:40
    for theta2=0:0.1:90
        for theta3=0:0.1:90
            fortheta4=0:0.1:20
        x=l1*cosd(theta1)+l2*cosd(theta1+theta2)+
l3*cosd(theta1+theta2+theta3)+
l4*cosd(theta1+theta2+theta3+theta4);
        y= l1*sind(theta1)+l2*sind(theta1+theta2)+
                l3*sind(theta1+theta2+theta3)+
                l4*sind(theta1+theta2+theta3+theta4);

plot(x,y,'r.');
            hold on;
            end
        end
    end
end
```

**Fig. 2.21**

```
a=40;
b=15;
for theta1=0:3:90
    for theta2=0:3:90
        for z=0:5:100
            x=a*cosd(theta1)+b*cosd(theta1+theta2);
            y=a*sind(theta1)+b*sind(theta1+theta2);
            plot3(x,y,z,'g.');
            hold on;
        end
    end
end
```

**Fig. 2.22–a**

```
l1=40;
l2=15;
l3=5;
c2=5;
c3=7;
fortheta1=0:1:90
    x=l1*cosd(theta1)+l2*cosd(theta1+theta1*sind(c2*t
    heta1))+
l3*cosd(theta1+theta1*sind(c2*theta1)+theta1*cosd(c3
*theta1));
y=l1*sind(theta1)+l2*sind(theta1+theta1*sind(c2*the
ta1))+
l3*sind(theta1+theta1*sind(c2*theta1)+theta1*cosd(c3
*theta1));
    plot(x,y,'r.');
    hold on;
end
```

**Fig. 2.22–b**

```
l1=40;
l2=15;
l3=5;
c2=3;
c3=2;
fortheta1=0:1:90
x=l1*cosd(theta1)+l2*cosd(theta1+theta1*sind(c2*t
heta1))+
l3*cosd(theta1+theta1*sind(c2*theta1)+theta1*cosd(c3
*theta1));
    y=l1*sind(theta1)+l2*sind(theta1+theta1*sind(c2*t
    heta1))+
l3*sind(theta1+theta1*sind(c2*theta1)+theta1*cosd(c3
*theta1));
    plot(x,y,'b.');
    hold on;
end
```

### Fig. 2.22-c

```
l1=40;
l2=15;
l3=5;
c2=3;
c3=4;
fortheta1=0:1:90
    x=l1*cosd(theta1)+l2*cosd(theta1+theta1*sind(c2*t
    heta1))+
l3*cosd(theta1+theta1*sind(c2*theta1)+theta1*cosd(c3
*theta1));
    y=l1*sind(theta1)+l2*sind(theta1+theta1*sind(c2*t
    heta1))+
l3*sind(theta1+theta1*sind(c2*theta1)+theta1*cosd(c3
*theta1));
    plot(x,y,'k.');
    hold on;
end
```

### Fig. 2.22-d

```
l1=40;
l2=15;
l3=5;
c2=-2;
c3=6;
fortheta1=0:1:90
    x=l1*cosd(theta1)+l2*cosd(theta1+theta1
    *sind(c2*theta1))+
l3*cosd(theta1+theta1*sind(c2*theta1)+theta1*co
sd(c3*theta1));
    y=l1*sind(theta1)+l2*sind(theta1+theta1
    *sind(c2*theta1))+
l3*sind(theta1+theta1*sind(c2*theta1)+theta1*co
sd(c3*theta1));
    plot(x,y,'g.');
    hold on;
end
```

**Fig. 2.22–e**

```
l1=40;
l2=15;
l3=5;
c2=-2;
c3=6;
fortheta1=0:0.1:40
   x=l1*cosd(theta1)+l2*cosd(theta1+theta1
   *tand(c2*theta1))+
l3*cosd(theta1+theta1*tand(c2*theta1)+theta1*co
sd(c3*theta1));
   y=l1*sind(theta1)+l2*sind(theta1+theta1
   *tand(c2*theta1))+
l3*sind(theta1+theta1*tand(c2*theta1)+theta1*co
sd(c3*theta1));
   plot(x,y,'c.');
   hold on;
end
```

**Fig. 2.22–f**

```
l1=40;
l2=15;
l3=5;
c2=-2;
c3=6;
fortheta1=0:0.1:40
      x=l1*cosd(theta1)+l2*cosd(theta1-
      theta1^(1/theta1))+
l3*cosd(theta1-theta1^(1/theta1)+theta1*cosd(c3
*theta1));
      y=l1*sind(theta1)+l2*sind(theta1-
      theta1^(1/theta1))+
l3*sind(theta1-theta1^(1/theta1)+theta1*cosd(c3
*theta1));
      plot(x,y,'y.');
      hold on;
end
```

# References


1. Alexander E, III, Maciunas RJ (1999). *Advanced Neurosurgical Navigation*. Thieme Medical, New York, pp. 333–338.
2. Allen BF, Jordan B, Pannell W, Lewis C, Dutson E, Faloutsos P (2010). Laparoscopic surgical robot for remote in vivo training, *Adv. Robot.*, **24**, 1679–1694.
3. Al-Niaimi AN, Einstein MH, Perry LT, Hartenbach EM, Kushner DM (2011). Uterine artery sparing robotic radical trachelectomy (AS-RRT) for early cancer of the cervix, *Int. J. Gynecol. Obstet.*, **112**, 76–80.
4. Argenziano M, Oz MC, Kohmoto T, Morgan J, Dimitui J, Mongero L, Beck J, Smith CR (2002). Totally endoscopic atrial septal defect repair with robotic assistance, *Heart Surg. Forum*, **5**, 194–297.
5. Asimov I, Frenkel K (1985). *Robots: Machines in Man's Image*. Harmony Books, New York, p. 19.
6. Asimov I, Retrieved November 07, 2012, from http://www.used-robots.com/robot-education.php?page=asimov.
7. Bann S, Khan M, Hernandez J, Munz Y, Moorthy K, Datta V, Rockall T, Darzi A (2003). Robotics in surgery, *J. Am. Coll. Surg.*, **196**(5), 784–795.
8. Bedini SA (Spring 1962). Thecompartmented cylindrical clepsydra, *Technol. Culture*, **3**(2), 115–141.
9. Bochkarev V, Ringley CD, Oleynikov D (2005). Robotic-assisted operative techniques in general surgery, *Oper. Tech. Gen. Surg.*, **7**(4), 188–200.
10. Bourla DH, Hubschman JP, Culjat M, Tsirbas A, Gupta A, Schwartz SD (2008). Feasibility study of intraocular robotic surgery with the da Vinci surgical system, *Retina*, **28**(1), 154–158.
11. Brandt G, Radermacher K, Zimolong A, Rau G, Merloz P, Klos TV, Robb J, Staudte HW (2000). CRIGOS: development of a compact robot for image-guided orthopedic surgery, *Orthopade*, **29**(7), 645–649.

12. Butner SE, Ghodoussi M (2003). Transforming a surgical robot for human telesurgery, *IEEE Trans. Robot. Autom.*, **19**(5), 818–824.
13. Cadeddu JA, Bzostek A, Schreiner S, Barnes AC, Roberts WW, Anderson JH, Taylor RH, Kavoussi LR (1997). A robotic system for percutaneous renal access, *J. Urol.*, **158**, 1589–1593.
14. Cadeire G, Himpens J, Vertruyen M, Favretti F (1999). The world's first obesity surgery performed by a surgeon at a distance, *Obes. Surg.*, **9**, 206–209.
15. Carpentier A, Loulmet D, Aupècle B, Kieffer JP, Tournay D, Guibourt P, Fiemeyer A, Méléard D, Richomme P, Cardon C (1998). Computer assisted open heart surgery: first case operated on with success, *C. R. Acad. Sci. III*, **321**, 437–442.
16. Casale P, Kojima Y (2009). Robotic-assisted laparoscopic surgery in pediatric urology: an update, *Scand. J. Surg.*, **98**, 110–119.
17. Cassilly R, Diodato M, Bottros M, Damiano RJ, Jr. (2004). Optimizing motion scaling and magnification in robotic surgery, *Surgery*, **136**(2), 291–294.
18. Castle SL, Kernstine KH (2008). Robotic-assisted thymectomy, *Sem. Thoracic Cardiovasc. Surg.*, **20**(4), 326–331.
19. Chan F, Kassim I, Lo C, Ho CL, Low D, Ang BT, Ng I (2009). Image-guided robotic neurosurgery: an in vitro and in vivo point accuracy evaluation experimental study, *Surg. Neurol.*, **71**, 640–648.
20. Chen W, Fu G, Gong J, He Y, Dong S (2002). A new design conception for large span deployable flat grid structures. *Int. J. Space Struct.*, **17**(4), 293–299.
21. Dalvand MM, Shirinzadeh B (2013). Motion control analysis of a parallel robot assisted minimally invasive surgery/microsurgery system (PRAMiSS), *Robot. Comput.-Integr. Manuf.*, **29**(2), 318–327.
22. Davies BL, Hibberd RD, Coptcoat MJ, Wickham JE (1989). A surgeon robot prostatectomy: a laboratory evaluation, *J. Med. Eng. Technol.*, **13**, 273–277.
23. Degueldre M, Vandromme J, Huong PT, Cadiere GB Robotically (2000). Assisted laparoscopic microsurgical tubal reanastomosis: a feasibility study, *Fertil. Steril.*, **74**, 1020–1023.
24. de Gennes PG, Okumura K, Shahinpoor M, Kim KJ (2000). Mechanoelectric effects in ionic gels, *Europhys. Lett.*, **50**(4), 513–518.
25. Del Grosso AE, Basso P (2010). Adaptive building skin structures, *Smart Mater. Struct.*, **19**(12), 124011.

26. Diaz-Arrastia C, Jurnalov C, Gomez G, Townsend C, Jr. (2002). Laparoscopic hysterectomy using a computer-enhanced surgical robot, *Surg. Endosc.*, **16**, 1271–1273.

27. Diodato M, Prasad S, Klingensmith M (2004). Robotics in surgery, *Curr. Probl. Surg.*, **41**, 752–810.

28. Diolaiti N (2010). Minimally invasive surgical system, US Patent No. 7725214.

29. Deole U, Lumia R, Shahinpoor M, Bermudez M (2008). Design and test of IPMC artificial muscle microgripper, *J. Micro-Nano Mechatron.*, Springer, Berlin, Heidelberg, doi:10.1007/s12213-008-0004-z.

30. Drasin T, Dutson E, Gracia C (2004). Use of a robotic system as surgical first assistant in advanced laparoscopic surgery, *J. Am. Coll. Surg.*, **199**(3), 368–373.

31. Fankhauser H, Glauser D, Flury P, Piguet Y, Epitaux M, Favre J, Meuli RA (1994). Robot for CT-guided stereotactic neurosurgery, *Stereotact. Funct. Neurosurg.*, **63**(1–4), 93–98.

32. Ferrara L, Shahinpoor M, Kim KJ, Schreyer B, Keshavarzi A, Benzel E, Lantz J (1999). Use of ionic polymer-metal composites (IPMCs) as a pressure transducer in the human spine, *Proc. SPIE Smart Materials and Structures Conference*, March 1-5, 1999, New Port Beach, California, Publication No. SPIE 3669-45, pp. 394–401.

33. Fest E, Shea K, Domer B, Smith IFC (2003). Adjustable tensegrity structures, *J. Struct. Eng.*, **129**(4), 515–526.

34. Gantes CJ, Konitopoulou E (2004). Geometric design of arbitrarily curved bistable deployable arches with discrete joint size. *Int. J. Solids Struct.*, **41**, 5517–5554.

35. Giorgi C, Sala R, Riva D, Cossu A, Eisenberg H (2000). Robotics in child neurosurgery, *Childs Nerv. Syst.*, **16**(10–11), 832–834.

36. Gomes P (2011). Surgical robotics: reviewing the past, analysing the present, imagining the future, *Robot. Comput.-Integr. Manuf.*, **27**(2), 261–266.

37. Guillonneau B, Jayet C, Tewari A, Vallancien G (2001). Robot assisted laparoscopic nephrectomy, *J. Urol.*, **166**, 200–201.

38. Haber GP, Crouzet S, Gill IS (2008). Laparoscopic and robotic assisted radical cystectomy for bladder cancer: a critical analysis, *Eur. Urol.*, **54**, 54–64.

39. Haidegger T, Benyo Z (2008). Surgical robotic support for long duration space missions, *Acta Astronaut.*, **63**, 996–1005.

40. Hemal AK, Menon M (2004). Robotics in urology, *Curr. Opin. Urol.*, **14**(2), 89–93.

41. Himpens J, Leman G, Cadiere GB (1998). Telesurgical laparoscopic cholecystectomy, *Surg. Endosc.*, **12**, 091.

42. Hoberman C (1990). Reversibly expandable doubly-curved truss structure, US Patent No. 4942700.

43. Hoberman C (1991). Radial expansion/retraction truss structures, US Patent No. 5024031.

44. Hoberman C (2007). *Unfolding Structures*, http://www.hoberman.com.

45. Horgan S, Vanuno D (2001). Robots in laparoscopic surgery, *J. Laparoendosc. Adv. Surg. Tech.*, **11**(6), 415–419.

46. Hoznek A, Zaki SK, Samadi DB, Salomon L, Lobontiu A, Lang P, Abbou CC (2002). Robotic assisted kidney transplantation: an initial experience, *J. Urol.*, **167**, 1604–1606.

47. Iordachita I, Kapoor A, Mitchell B, Kazanzides P, Hager G, Handa J, Taylor R (2006). *Steady-Hand Manipulator for Retinal Surgery*. Johns Hopkins University.

48. Jakopec M, Harris SJ, Rodriguez y Baena F, Gomes P, Cobb J, Davies BL (2001). The first clinical application of a "hands-on" robotic knee surgery system, *Comput.-Aided Surg.*, **6**, 329–339.

49. Kaiser WA, Fischer H, Vagner J, Selig M (2000). Robotic system for biopsy and therapy of breast lesions in a high-field whole-body magnetic resonance tomography unit, *Invest. Radiol.*, **35**, 513–519.

50. Kassabian P, You Z, Pellegrino S (1999). Retractable roof structures, *Proc. Inst. Civil Eng. Struct. Build.*, **134**, 45–56.

51. Keshavarzi A, Shahinpoor M, Kim, KJ, Lantz J (1999). Blood pressure, pulse rate, and rhythm measurement using ionic polymer-metal composites sensors, *Proc. SPIE Smart Materials and Structures Conference*, March 1-5, 1999, New Port Beach, California, Publication No. SPIE 3669-36, pp. 369–376.

52. Kim KJ, Shahinpoor M (2005). A novel method of manufacturing three-dimensional ionic polymer-metal composites (IPMC's) biomimetic sensors, actuators and artificial muscle, *Polymer*, **43**(3), 797–802.

53. Koren Y (1985). *Robotics for Engineers*. McGraw & Hill.

54. Kwoh YS, Hou J, Jonckheere EA, Hayati S (1988). A robot with improved absolute positioning accuracy for CT guided stereotactic brain surgery, *IEEE Trans. Biomed. Eng.*, **35**, 153–160.

55. Kypson AP, Nifong LW, Chitwood WR, Jr. (2003). Robotic cardiac surgery, *J. Long-Term Eff. Med. Implants*, **13**(6), 451–464.

56. Larkin DQ, Shafer DC (2011). Robotic surgery system including position sensors using fiber Bragg gratings, US Patent No. 7930065.

57. Le Roux PD, Das H, Esquenazi S, Kelly PJ (2001). Robot-assisted microsurgery: a feasibility study in the rat, *Neurosurgery*, **48**, 584–589.

58. Lum MJH, Rosen J, Lendvay TS, Wright AS, Sinanan MN, Hannaford B (2008). TeleRobotic fundamentals of laparoscopic surgery (FLS): effects of time delay-pilot study, *Conf. Proc. IEEE Eng. Med. Biol. Soc.*, **2008**, 5597–5600.

59. Ma J, Berkelman P (2007). Task evaluations of a compact laparoscopic surgical robot system, *IEEE/RSJ Int. Conf. Intell. Robots Syst., IROS 2007*, October 29–November 2, 2007.

60. Maden F, Korkmaza K, Akgünb Y (2011). A review of planar scissor structural mechanisms: geometric principles and design methods, *Archit. Sci. Rev.*, **54**(3), 246–257.

61. Malone R (1978). *The Robot Book*. Push Pin Press, New York, p. 26.

62. Mao SP, Lai HC, Chang FW, Yu MH, Chang CC (2007). Laparoscopy-assisted robotic myomectomy using the da Vinci system, *Taiwan J. Obstet. Gynecol.*, **46**(2), 174–176.

63. Marescaux J, Smith MK, Fölscher D, Jamali F, Malassagne B, Leroy J (2001). Telerobotic laparoscopic cholecystectomy: initial experience with 25 patients, *Ann. Surg.*, **234**, 1–7.

64. Margossian H, Garcia-Ruiz A, Falcone T, Goldberg JM, Attaran M, Gagner M (1998). Robotically assisted laparoscopic microsurgical uterine horn anastomosis, *Fertil. Steril.*, **70**, 530–534.

65. Martinez BD, Wiegand CS (2004). Robotics in vascular surgery, *Am. J. Surg.*, **188**(Suppl to October 2004), 57S–62S.

66. Meenink HCM, Hendrix R, Rosielle PCJN, Steinbuch M, Nijmeijer H, de Smet MC (2010). A master-μslave robot for vitreo-retinal eye surgery, *Proc. Euspen Int. Conf.*, Delft.

67. Micali S, Virgili G, Vannozzi E, Grassi N, Jarrett TW, Bauer JJ, Vespasiani G, Kavoussi LR (2000). Feasibility of telementoring between Baltimore (USA) and Rome (Italy): the first five cases, *J. Endourol.*, **14**, 493–496.

68. Mirbagheri A, Farahmand F, Meghdari A, Karimian F (2011). Design and development of an effective low cost robotic cameraman for laparoscopic surgery: RoboLens, Sci. Iran., **18**(1), 105–114.

69. Mitchell B, Koo J, Iordachita I, Kazanzides P, Kapoor A, Handa J, Hager G, Taylor R (2007). Development and application of a new steady-hand manipulator for retinal surgery, *2007 IEEE Int. Conf. Robot. Autom. (Roma, Italy)*, April 10–14, 2007.
70. Mohr FW, Falk V, Diegeler A, Autschback R (1999). Computer-enhanced coronary artery bypass surgery, *J. Thorac. Cardiovasc. Surg.*, **117**, 1212–1214.
71. Munz Y, Moorthy K, Kudchadkar R, Hernandez JD, Martin S, Darzi A, Rockall T (2004). Robotic assisted rectopexy, *Am. J. Surg.*, **187**, 88–92.
72. Ng WS, Davies BL, Hibberd RD, Timoney AG (1993). A firsthand experience in transurethral resection of the prostate, *IEEE EMBS J.*, **1993**, 123–125.
73. Nowlin WC, Mohr PW, Schena BM, Larkin DQ, Guthart G (2011). Software center and highly configurable robotic systems for surgery and other uses, US Patent No. 8004229.
74. Olsen LH (2006). Robotics in pediatric urology, *J. Pediatr. Urol.*, **2**, 40e45, Education article.
75. Onnasch JF, Schneider F, Falk V, Mierzwa M, Bucerius J, Mohr FW (2002). Five years of less invasive minimal surgery: from experimental to routine, *Heart Surg. Forum*, **5**, 132–135.
76. Onoda J, Fu D-Y, Minesugi K (1996). Two-dimensional deployable hexapod truss, *J. Spacecraft Rockets*, **33**, 416–421.
77. Patel K (2008). Robotics the future of surgery, *Int. J. Surg.*, **6**, 441–442.
78. Patel MN, Menon M, Rogers CG (2010). Robotic partial nephrectomy: a comparison to current techniques, *Urol. Oncol.: Sem. Original Invest.*, **28**, 74–76, seminar article.
79. Pellegrino S, Calladine CR (1986). Matrix analysis of statically and kinematically indeterminate frameworks, *Int. J. Solids Struct.*, **22**, 409–402.
80. Pinero EP (1961). Project for a mobile theatre, *Archit. Des.*, **12**, 570.
81. Pires NJ (2000). Using actual industrial robot manipulators with construction tasks, *Proc. 17th ISARC*, Taipei, Taiwan, 1–5.
82. Prasad SM, Maniar HS, Soper NJ, Damiano RJ, Jr., Klingensmith ME (2002). The effect of robotic assistance on learning curves for basic laparoscopic skills, *Am. J. Surg.*, **183**, 702–707.
83. Prasad SM, Maniar HS, Chu C, Schuessler RB, Damiano RJ, Jr. (2004). Surgical robotics: impact of motion scaling on task performance, *J. Am. Coll. Surg.*, **199**(6), 863–868.
84. Rosheim ME (1994). *Robot Evolution: The Development of Anthrobotics*. John Wiley and Sons, p. 2.

85. Sabharwal A, Pradhan S, Kumar A (2006). Current role of robotics in urology, *Apollo Med.*, **3**(4), 365–370.

86. Shahinpoor M (1996). Multifingered grabbers as smart structures for robotic applications, *Proc. SPIE 2779*, **1000**.

87. Shahinpoor M (2000). Ion-exchange membrane-metal composite as biomimetic sensors and actuators, in *Polymer Sensors and Actuators* (eds. Osada Y, De Rossi D). Springer-Verlag, Heidelberg, pp. 325–359.

88. Shahinpoor M (2002). Artificial muscles, in *Encyclopedia of Biomaterials and Biomedical Engineering* (eds. Wnek G, Bowlin G). Marcel Dekker, New York, pp. 43–52.

89. Shahinpoor M (2003). Ionic polymer-conductor composites as biomimetic sensors, robotic actuators and artificial muscles: a review, *Electrochim. Acta*, **48**(14–16), 2343–2353.

90. Shahinpoor M (2005). Soft plastic robots and artificial muscles, *Int. J. Adv. Robot. Syst.*, **2**(2), 161–174.

91. Shahinpoor M (2008). Ionic polymeric conductor nano composites (IPCMCs) as distributed nanosensors and nanoactuators, *Adv. Sci. Technol. J.*, **54**, 70–81, Trans Tech, Switzerland.

92. Shahinpoor M (2009). Biomimetics nananosensors and nanoactuators, in Biomimetics and *Bioinspired Nanomaterials*, Vol. 7 (eds. Challa SS, Kumar R). John Wiley and Sons, Wiley-VCH Verlag, GmnH & Co. KGaA, Weinheim, Germany, pp. 1–26.

93. Shahinpoor M (2009). Recent advances in ionic polymer metal nanocomposites as distributed biomimetic nanosensors, nanoactuators and artificial muscles, *J. Phys., CS 127* (2008–2009).

94. Shahinpoor M (2011). *Intelligent Robotic Systems: Modeling & Simulation*, 2nd ed. ERI Press, Albuquerque, New Mexico.

95. Shahinpoor M, Gheshmi S (2012). Space-Saving Laparoscopic Surgical Slave Robot, US Provisional Patent Application No. 61718822, November, 2012.

96. Shahinpoor M, Gheshmi S, Soltanpour D (2012). Intraocular robotic surgical system, US Provisional Patent Application No. 61716718, December, 2012.

97. Shahinpoor M, Kim KJ (2002). A solid-state soft actuator exhibiting large electromechanical effect, *Appl. Phys. Lett.*, **80**(18), 3445–3447.

98. Shahinpoor M, Kim KJ (2005). Ionic polymer-metal composites: iv industrial and medical applications (Review paper), *Smart Mater. Struct.* **14**(1), 197–214.

99. Shahinpoor M, Kim KJ, Mojarrad M (2007). *Artificial Muscles: Applications of Advanced Polymeric Nano-Composites*. CRC Press, Taylor and Francis, London, New York.

100. Shahinpoor M, Schneider HJ (2008). Intelligent Materials, 1st ed. Royal Society of Chemistry (RSC) Cambridge, Great Britain.

101. Shew SB, Ostlie DJ, Holcomb GW, III (2003). Robotic telescopic assistance in pediatric laparoscopic surgery, *Pediatr. Endosurg. Innovative Tech.*, **7**(4).

102. Siwek LG, Reynolds B (2007). Totally robotic mitral valve repair, *Oper. Tech. Thoracic Cardiovasc. Surg.*, **12**(4), 235–249.

103. Sofla A, Elzey D, Wadley H (2009). Shape morphing hinged truss structures, *Smart Mater. Struct.*, **18**, 065012.

104. Strong M (2004). Protein nanomachines, *PLOS Biol.*, **2**, 0305.

105. Sutherland GR, Louw DF, McBeth PB, Fielding T, Gregoris DJ (2006). Microsurgical robot system, US Patent No. 7155316, December 26, 2006.

106. Sutherland GR, Louw DF, McBeth PB, Fielding T, Gregoris DJ (2012). Microsurgical robot system, US Patent No. 8170717, May 1, 2012.

107. Sweeney T, Rattner DW (2002). Robotically assisted minimally invasive biliary surgery in a porcine model, *Surg. Endosc.*, **16**, 138–141.

108. Taylor RH, Stoianovici D (2003). Medical robotics in computer-integrated surgery, *IEEE Trans. Robot. Autom.*, **19**(5), 765–781.

109. Tchartchian G, Dietzel J, Bojahr B, Hackethal A, De Wilde R (2011). Decreasing strain on the surgeon in gynecologic minimally invasive surgery by using semi-active robotics, *Int. J. Gynecol. Obstet.*, **112**, 72–75.

110. Terris DJ, Amin SH (2008). Robotic and endoscopic surgery in the neck, *Oper. Tech. Otolaryngol: Head Neck Surg.*, **19**(1), 36–41.

111. Tesla N (1898). Method of and apparatus for controlling mechanism of moving vessels of vehicles, US Patent No. 613809, November 8, 1898.

112. Tewari A, Peabody J, Sarle R, Balakrishnan G, Hemal A, Shrivastava A, Menon M (2002). Technique of da Vinci robot-assisted anatomic radical prostatectomy, *Urology*, **60**, 569–572.

113. Torraca L, Ismeno G, Quarti A, Alfieri O (2002). Totally endoscopic atrial septal defect closure with a robotic system: experience with seven cases, *Heart Surg. Forum*, **5**, 125–127.

114. Tsirbas A, Mango C, Dutson E (2007). Use of robotics for intraocular surgery, robotic ocular surgery, *Br. J. Ophthalmol.*, **91**(1), 18–21.

115. Tsui I, Tsirbas A, Mango CW, Schwartz SD, Hubschman JP (2010). *Robotic Surgery in Ophthalmology* (ed. Baik SH).InTech, ISBN: 978-953-7619-77-0.

116. Tsutomu K, Tokai H (1997). Cable scissors arch-marionettic structure. structural morphology, towards the new millennium, *Proc. Int. Conf. of IASS*, 107–116, University of Nottingham.

117. Ueta T, Yamaguchi Y, Shirakawa Y, Nakano T, Ideta R, Noda Y, Morita A, Mochizuki R, Sugita N, Mitsuishi M, Tamaki Y (2009). Robot-assisted vitreoretinal surgery: development of a prototype and feasibility studies in an animal model, **116**(8), 1538.e2–1543.e2.

118. Van Der Brug WP, De Bliek HLT, Gerritsen FA (1999). Image-guided surgery system, US Patent No. 6006127.

119. White MA, Haber GP, Autorino R, Khanna R, Forest S, Yang B, Altunrende F, Stein RJ, Kaouk JH (2010). Robotic laparoendoscopic single-site radical prostatectomy: technique and early outcomes, *Eur. Urol.*, **58**, 544–550.

120. Wisselink W, Cuesta MA, Gracia C, Rauwerda JA (2002). Robot-assisted laparoscopic aortobifemoral bypass for aortoiliac occlusive disease: a report of two cases, *J. Vasc. Surg.*, 2002;36:1079–1082.

121. Yildrim Y (1010). *Cytoreductive Surgery in Gynecologic Oncology: A Multidisciplinary Approach.* Transworld Research Network, Kerala, India, pp. 213–232.

# Author Index

# Subject Index